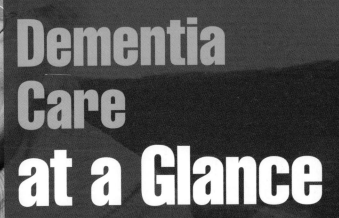

Dementia Care at a Glance

Catharine Jenkins

School of Nursing, Midwifery and Social Work Professions
Faculty of Health Education and Life Sciences
Birmingham City University
Birmingham, UK

Laura Ginesi

School of Nursing Sciences
Faculty of Medicine and Health Sciences
University of East Anglia
Norwich, UK

Bernie Keenan

School of Nursing, Midwifery and Social Work Professions
Faculty of Health Education and Life Sciences
Birmingham City University
Birmingham, UK

Series editor: Ian Peate

WILEY Blackwell

This edition first published 2016 © 2016 by John Wiley & Sons Ltd.

Registered office: John Wiley & Sons, Ltd, The Atrium, Southern Gate, Chichester, West Sussex, PO19 8SQ, UK

Editorial offices: ~~9600 Garsington Road, Oxford, OX4 2DQ, UK~~

The Atrium, Southern Gate, Chichester, West Sussex, PO19 8SQ, UK

350 Main Street, Malden, MA 02148-5020, USA

For details of our global editorial offices, for customer services and for information about how to apply for permission to reuse the copyright material in this book please see our website at www.wiley.com/wiley-blackwell

Library of Congress Cataloging-in-Publication Data

Jenkins, Catharine, 1960– , author.
  Dementia care at a glance / Catharine Jenkins, Laura Ginesi, Bernie Keenan.
    p. ; cm. — (At a glance series)
  Includes bibliographical references and index.
  ISBN 978-1-118-85998-8 (pbk.)
  I. Ginesi, Laura, 1956– , author.   II. Keenan, Bernie, 1957– , author.
III. Title.   IV. Series: At a glance series (Oxford, England)
  [DNLM: 1. Dementia.   2. Caregivers.   3. Patient Care—methods. WM 220]
  RC521
  616.8'3—dc23

                          2015010258

A catalogue record for this book is available from the British Library.

Wiley also publishes its books in a variety of electronic formats. Some content that appears in print may not be available in electronic books.

Cover image: Courtesy of the authors

Set in Minion Pro 9.5/11.5 by Aptara

Printed and bound in Singapore by Markono Print Media Pte Ltd

1   2016

Contents

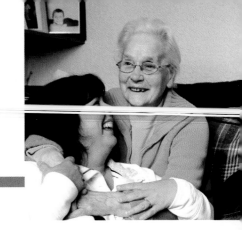

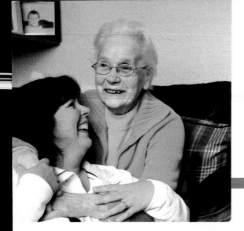

Preface

People who have dementia, their family members and friends, care assistants, professionals in training, those with long experience in the field, people who interact with the public in order to provide a product or service and those who want to contribute to dementia-friendly communities – all have a part to play in dementia care. The aim of this book is to empower people supporting others who are living with dementia, so that professional and family carer roles are more enjoyable and rewarding and so that the lives of those living with dementia are more secure, more fun and more meaningful. The book sets about achieving this aim by placing the experience of the person with dementia in the centre, highlighting the impact of individuals, society and the physical environment on the person's life.

Dementia is a 'hot topic', with headlines in the media about the 'rising tide' of older people and the cost of the dementia-related consequences of these demographic changes. Reports about poor quality of care in residential and nursing homes or abuse of vulnerable older people also makes headlines that can be a source of worry for those who are concerned about their family members and/or thinking about how they would like to be looked after in old age. These headlines ignore the good quality care that is the norm for most people.

We feel that excellence in dementia care is 'everybody's business' because the disease can affect people from every sector of society. Our approach is based on the belief that everyone can benefit from an inclusive approach. We recognise that people with dementia and their supporters live in a wider context of social networks and physical environments, so the book aims to offer guidance on achievable initiatives and adjustments that make a difference to continued inclusion of people with dementia in their communities.

This book is designed to be an introductory text so it includes key facts and information essential for insight into the nature of the difficulties associated with dementia and of approaches that make a positive difference to well-being. Recognising that people with dementia have a lot to offer others, we highlight the importance of mutual support and adopt a challenging approach to stigma and exclusion; we try to offer alternatives and solutions to societal as well as individual problems.

Specialist skills may be both 'invisible' and internalised. Workers and family carers may be experts in their roles yet receive little recognition because their abilities look 'natural' to an observer. Empathy – the ability to put yourself in another person's shoes – and kindness are the basis of excellent care and can minimise stress for people with dementia. We hope to make knowledge and skills explicit and hope to clarify what needs to be done to create positive outcomes for people who have dementia. In sharing our experience of caring for people with dementia in different hospital, community and home environments, we aim to acknowledge challenges while offering guidance in an engaging, informative, encouraging and accessible way. Improved knowledge, better understanding and specific advice based on years of experience can be applied by anyone involved in procedures or social care interventions and promote positive outcomes.

We have tried to approach dementia care holistically, so that all aspects of life are considered and all groups in society included. We believe that the well-being of those involved in care – either as family or paid carers – is as important as that of the person with dementia. We take a person-centred approach that respects the needs of all involved. This book is an introduction for developing professionals of all backgrounds, but it is equally relevant for family carers and people with a diagnosis of dementia themselves. With earlier diagnoses people with dementia need access to clear honest explanations of issues that can affect them at different stages of the 'dementia journey' and of the effective services and interventions available.

The book is organised into parts to make it easier for the reader to navigate and to follow their interests. We begin by outlining the context and how the various types of dementia are caused and how they progress. Following this we order the chapters to reflect the progression of dementia, from reducing risk and health promotion, through relationship and diversity issues, potential problems and a wide range of potential responses, to ethical and legal issues and considering future developments. Throughout the book we encourage an empathic sensitive and person-centred approach.

The structure is designed to make the book accessible to a wide range of readers who may be using it in a variety of different locations, including hospital wards, voluntary sector organisations, colleges and universities and in the community in respite or day care centres and in people's own homes. It will also be useful for those wishing to revise the subject and reinforce learning for specific events such as job interviews and examinations.

The book offers an in-depth introduction that will develop and embed learning. Further reading is signposted at the end of the book. An online resource is available which challenges the reader with ideas for reflective writing and a quiz to promote and reinforce learning.

We thank our readers for their interest and commitment to the care of people with dementia. We hope that this book will be helpful in supporting you in your work promoting the well-being of those in your care. We thank the people with dementia who have contributed to our own learning and aim now to pass this on to our readers.

Acknowledgements

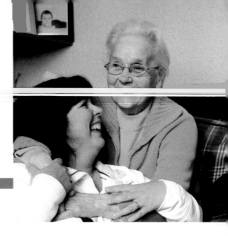

With thanks to: Mrs. McNeil, her daughter Margaret and all families living with dementia. Your commitment, patience, humour and resourcefulness through the difficulties of living with dementia have inspired us to write this book.

The Royal Star and Garter Home, Solihull, for allowing photography of their person-centred and stimulating care environment.

Our families, for your encouragement and support.

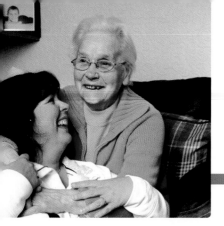

About the companion website

Do not forget to visit the companion website for this book:

www.ataglanceseries.com/nursing/
dementiacare

There you will find valuable material designed to enhance
your learning, including:

- Interactive multiple choice questions
- Reflective questions

Scan this QR code to visit the companion website

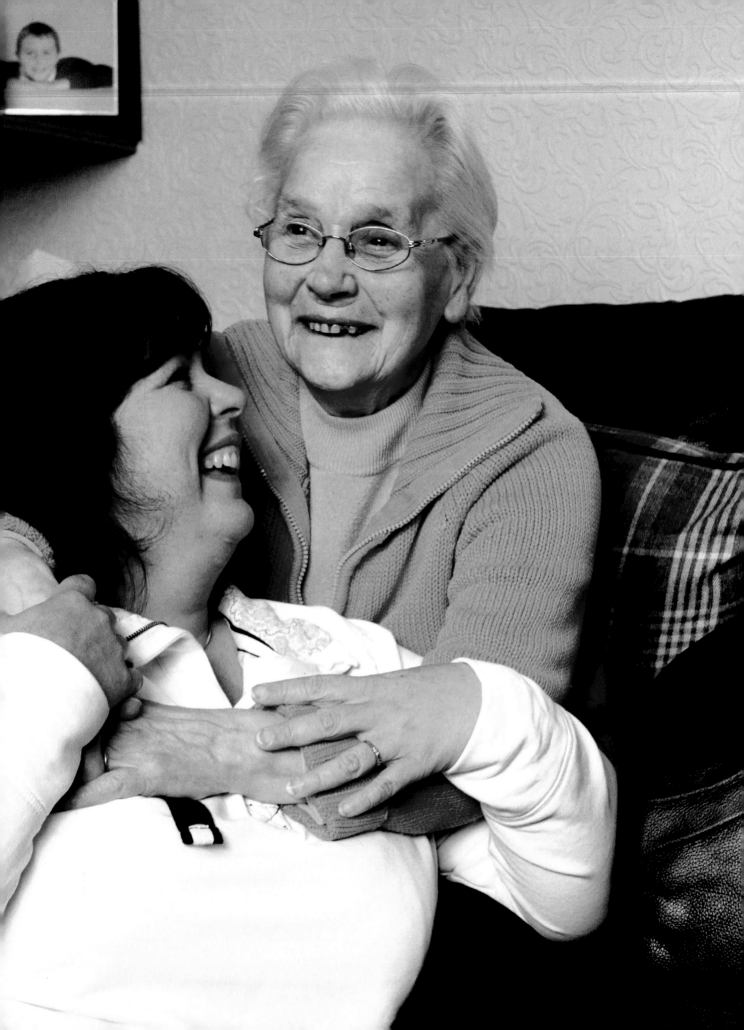

Setting the scene

Part 1

Chapters

1 Introduction

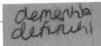

Figure 1.1 Dementia facts

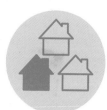

1/3 of people with dementia live on their own in the community

However, only 23% of people think it is possible for people with dementia to live on their own

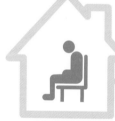

62%

of people with dementia living alone feel lonely

38%

of people with dementia feel lonely

24%

of over 55s have felt lonely in the last month

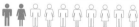

Source: http://www.alzheimers.org.uk/infographic
Reproduced with permission of the Alzheimer's Society

Context

'Dementia' is an umbrella term, referring to a range of conditions associated with old age ~~which~~ ~~language skills~~ cognitive functioning and the ability to carry out everyday activities of daily living are progressively weakened due to processes within the brain that lead to gradual neuronal death. Dementia is not a natural part of ageing, and most older people do not develop dementia. However, for those who are affected, it has an impact on their ability to be independent, to engage with others as equals, to look after everyday basic needs and to maintain usual roles in society. Some of these consequences are related to the stigma still associated with dementia rather than the actual condition itself. Relationships are central to the well-being of people with dementia, yet sometimes friends and relatives do not feel able to interact with and support loved ones, which can lead to feelings of isolation (Figure 1.1).

Demographic factors mean that ever larger numbers of people are expected to be living with dementia in the near future. Therefore, there is a pressing need to let people know what they can do to minimise stigma, to understand the disease processes and their impact, to communicate effectively and to play a part in changing relationships, society and the physical environment so that we welcome and include those living with dementia. At the same time, current and future generations can learn how to minimise the risk of developing dementia by making simple lifestyle adjustments.

Who the book is for

In this context, people with dementia, their family members, health and social care professionals, student nurses and other professionals in training, voluntary workers and concerned members of communities need information about dementia, insight into people's experiences and guidance on appropriate support and interventions. This book is for anyone in these situations who wants to make a positive difference to the experiences of people living with dementia.

Overview of dementia

There are many types of dementia; the most frequently occurring are Alzheimer's disease (60–70% of cases) and vascular dementia. Other forms include Lewy body disease, mixed dementia (Alzheimer's combined with vascular-type pathology), frontotemporal dementia, posterior cortical atrophy, alcohol-related dementia and Creutzfeldt–Jakob disease. While these conditions differ in their causation, specific patterns of development and initial symptomatology, they have much in common. All affect short-term memory, emotions, cognition, language and the ability to sequence activities and so cope with everyday life. We outline the most common types of dementia in the early chapters and subsequently use the term 'dementia' to cover all forms.

Defining our terms

'Dementia' is used to refer to the conditions outlined previously. The people who have a form of dementia are called 'people with dementia' or 'people living with dementia' throughout the book. This is because dementia does not, and should not, eliminate the person – we feel it is useful to separate the condition so that it is reinforced that despite its effects, these do not overwhelm the history, personality, lifetime experiences and relationships of a person.

'Stages' of dementia

All forms of dementia are progressive, which means they gradually get worse. We refer to dementia developing in stages, although in reality the stages ~~described~~ ~~... a~~ neat pattern, as each individual's experience is unique. 'Early stages' means those who may have recently had concerns about memory confirmed and those who may have come to terms with their diagnosis and are continuing to live independently, despite some problems with short-term memory and word-finding difficulties. People in this situation can usually continue to drive and continue with their social roles, although professional life may be difficult. They may wish to let other people know of their diagnosis, so as to explain any problems that might arise (such as forgetting names, getting lost in unfamiliar environments), and may need a little support but are generally able to articulate their wishes and carry them out. As time goes on, people living with dementia may experience further difficulties, for example, risks related to forgetting to turn gas or taps off, difficulties expressing themselves, problem-solving or following TV programmes. They may need prompting with some activities of daily living and at times may need assistance. Later on, people may struggle to live independently and find it difficult to understand other people and to express their own thoughts and feelings. In later stages, they will need more assistance with simple tasks. Life can become frustrating, particularly when others do not understand and make adjustments. Family carers can find caring very stressful. All forms of dementia are terminal conditions and grow similar in later stages. Eventually the person will need palliative care (care aiming to keep a person comfortable and pain free at end of life).

Causes for optimism

Despite the negative prognosis, there is much that can be done to improve well-being for those living with dementia and to anticipate in treatment breakthroughs in the future. Funding for research is at its highest levels ever and more money is committed. Anti-dementia drugs have some positive effects and new drugs are being trialled. Many countries have national strategies outlining the importance of high-quality care, support and social inclusion throughout the condition. Campaigns to eradicate stigma are already making a difference to peoples' lives and architects are becoming more aware of how dementia-friendly environments can promote independence.

The strengths of people with dementia

People with dementia themselves are increasingly confident about talking about their condition and campaigning for change by blogging, addressing conferences and contributing to government policy development.

Our beliefs and approach

We take the view that people living with dementia are valuable citizens and that it is everybody's business to ensure they are supported so as to have the best quality of life. This means addressing social inclusion, optimum physical health and a range of interventions, treatments and therapies. The experiences of people with dementia result mainly from the quality of relationships, so most of all we hope to promote positive, person-centred interpersonal connections.

2 The experiences of people with dementia

Figure 2.1 The artwork of William Utermohlen

William Utermohlen was an artist who continued to paint and draw throughout his condition. His work illustrates his changing sense of self

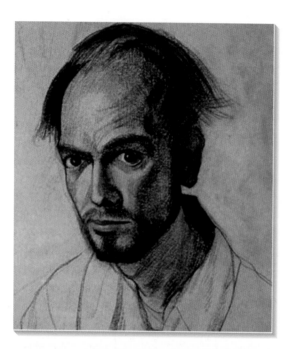
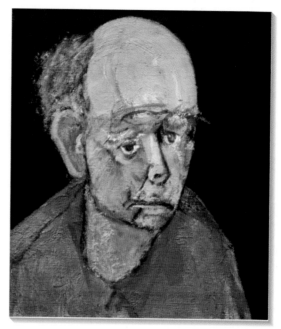
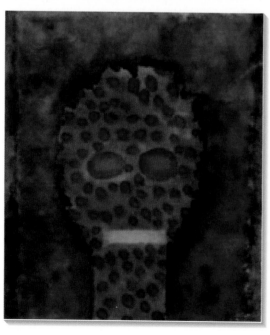
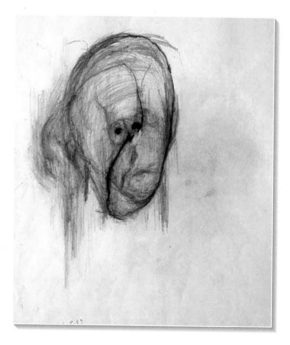

Source: *Reproduced with permission of Chris Boïcos Fine Arts, Paris*

Dementia Care at a Glance, First Edition. Catharine Jenkins, Laura Ginesi and Bernie Keenan. © 2016 by John Wiley & Sons, Ltd. Published 2016 by John Wiley & Sons, Ltd.
Companion website: www.ataglanceseries.com/nursing/dementiacare

Gaining insight into people's experiences

In the early stages of dementia, people are able to describe their experiences, thoughts and feelings. As the dementia progresses, this

The experience of having dementia is unique and very personal. Even though there is a general pattern in how the syndromes progress, each person's journey will be different because of other factors such as their personality, the type of dementia, the nature of their close relationships and support network, educational level, economic situation and location. In addition, dementia is still often stigmatised and awareness of having a 'damaged identity' plays a part in an individual's sense of self.

Professionals and family members wishing to gain insight into the world and experience of a person with dementia, therefore, need to listen closely and sensitively to how the person communicates about what it is like to live with the condition. They can also attempt to gain insight through other means and empathise by imagining how they might feel if they had the difficulties associated with dementia.

Listening to people with dementia

The most effective way to find out about someone's experience is to ask them. A question such as 'what's it like living with your condition?', should enable a person in early or middle stages of dementia to open up about how they feel and what their life involves. It is important to listen patiently and be aware that the person may use metaphors to describe the situation and these may not obviously or immediately answer the question. Observational skills will enable a sensitive person to read the mood of the person with dementia who in later stages may not be able to express thoughts coherently. 'Reading between the lines' can allow some understanding. For example, the person with dementia may be feeling uneasy, frightened or disorientated, so he/she might talk about being in a strange place or ask for clues about where they are or who is talking to them.

People living with dementia are experts about their own experiences and increasingly they are taking the initiative in sharing their insights. The most famous of these was Terry Pratchett, who spoke on radio and TV, while Christine Bryden wrote *Dancing with Dementia* (2005). Some people with dementia (e.g. Norm McNamara) have also taken to blogging and have created websites (e.g. Jennifer Bute).

Learning through creative media

Literature, films and works of art can also contribute to an understanding of people's experiences. *Still Alice* (Genova, 2009) and *The Story of Forgetting* (Block, 2009) explore the issues as do the films 'Iris', about the life of author Iris Murdoch, and 'The Iron Lady', about former Prime Minister Margaret Thatcher. William Utermohlen's art illustrates his changing awareness of self during the course of his illness (Figure 2.1).

Stigma

In many people's minds, dementia is associated with decline and death, leading to fear and denial that these experiences could

and feelings, so they attempt to put them, and those that remind them that old age comes to us all, to one side, out of sight and mind.

There is a long-standing history of excluding people with dementia from wider society, reinforced by labelling their disabilities as signs of being 'less alive' or less of a person. Naturally this leads to a fear in the mind of a forgetful person who, as a member of the same society, has internalised these values. Any sign of a poor memory can be perceived as the beginning of loss of social self as well as personal identity.

Knowing this, people with dementia are faced with the difficult decision about whether to be open about their condition and thus contribute to dismantling prejudice, or try to maintain their sense of self and self-esteem despite insensitivity and discrimination within society. Kitwood (1997) called undermining responses to people with dementia 'malignant social psychology' (Chapter 15). The term reflects the extent of the damage that can be done when stigma and beliefs drive behaviour that limits and damages people's opportunities and relationships.

Recent initiatives such as the 'Dementia Challenge' (Alzheimer's Society, 2012) and 'Dementia Friends' in the United Kingdom aim to reverse this thinking and maintain people with dementia as citizens within their societies while enabling adjustments to be made to ensure they maintain their roles, with support if necessary, in their families and communities.

Memory and identity

Our memories allow us to reinforce our identities through individual stories that remind us what we have done and the values and relationships that sustain an identity. Losing recent memories and having difficulty in thinking coherently threatens this process. People with dementia sometimes express a feeling of struggling in a fog to understand and communicate. Long-term intact memories gradually become more real than recent or current events. Difficulty with managing tasks and a lack of understanding from others can give rise to anger and frustration. Embarrassment and feelings of inadequacy arise when someone is reminded of their deficits. They may also fear how their worsening condition could make them a burden on family members. Feelings of sadness are common while a mood may persist when the trigger that caused it has been forgotten. Emotional responses remain strong and the experience of a person in later stages is dependent on the nature of close relationships and the willingness of family members and professional carers to promote identity and well-being through meaningful activities, emotional warmth and social inclusion.

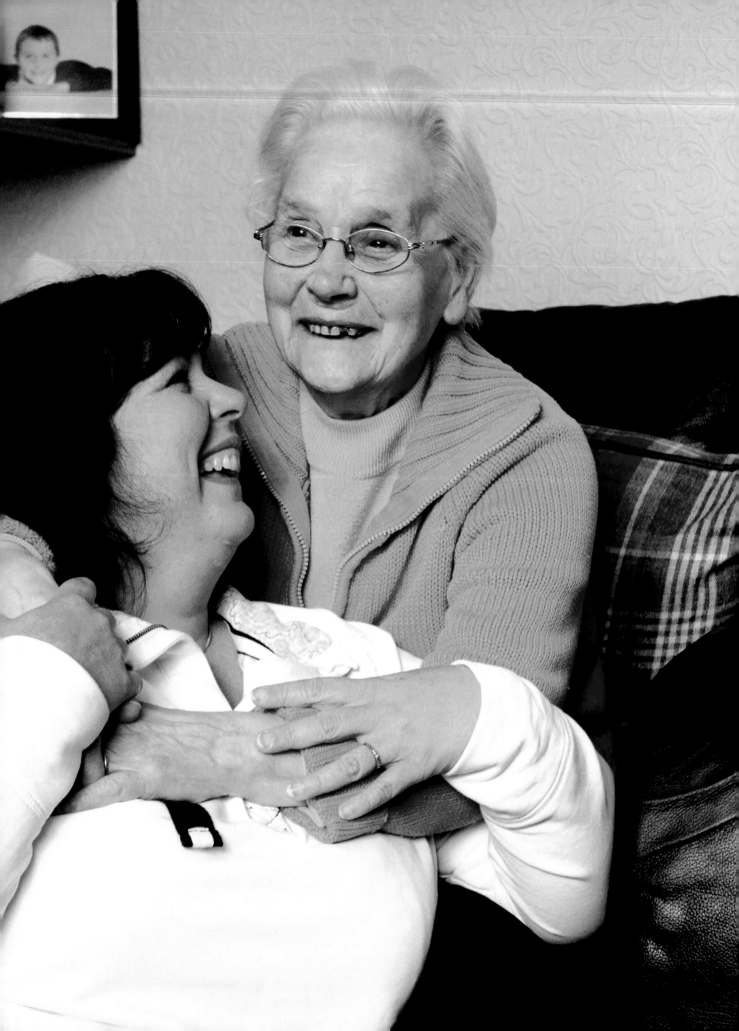

Dementia causes and types

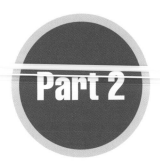

Chapters

3 Brain basics

Figure 3.1 Human nervous system

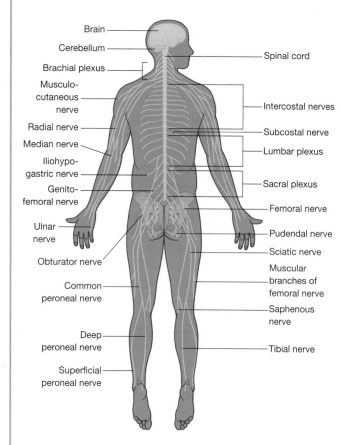

Figure 3.3a Cerebral cortex

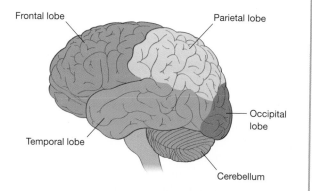

Figure 3.3b The limbic cortex is located within the cerebral cortex

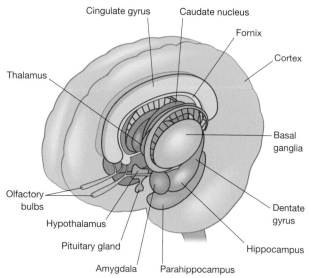

Figure 3.2 Divisions of the nervous system

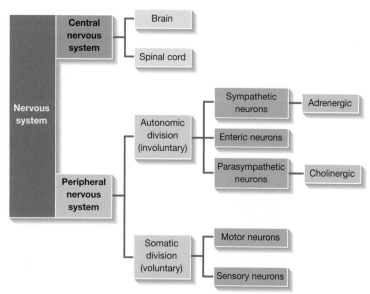

Figure 3.4 How neurons are classified

Neurons are classified according to:

- The type of fibres (axons and dendrites)
- The function of the neuron (sensory or motor)
- The type and nature of synaptic connection(s) formed with other neurons (excitatory or inhibitory)
- The type of neurotransmitter molecule secreted from their terminal (e.g. adrenergic, cholinergic or dopaminergic)

Some release neurohormones (e.g. oxytocin and adrenalin) or other signal molecules including nitric oxide

Source: Benedict Campbell/ Wellcome Images

Dementia Care at a Glance, First Edition. Catharine Jenkins, Laura Ginesi and Bernie Keenan. © 2016 by John Wiley & Sons, Ltd. Published 2016 by John Wiley & Sons, Ltd.
Companion website: www.ataglanceseries.com/nursing/dementiacare

Introduction to the brain

The human nervous system (Figure 3.1) is both crucial for life and responsible for sensation, movement, thought and speech. The adult brain, which weighs 1.3–1.4 kg, has been likened to an information-processing unit like a computer because it receives sensory information, integrates it and coordinates a behavioural response. In reality, the brain is much more complex than a machine because of its ability to generate information and responses in the absence of external input. Dementia is an umbrella term for about 100 diseases in which brain cells die on a large scale. It can help to know about key structures and regions of the brain because the progressive degeneration affects many cognitive functions – memory, attention, problem-solving, mental agility, language, perception, emotion and planning.

The nervous system

Estimates of the number of cells in the nervous system vary but it is thought to comprise 100 billion **neurons** (nerve cells) and support tissue (known as **neuroglia** or glia). Neurons are called physiologically excitable cells because they are able to conduct electrical impulses (action potentials) that enable rapid communication. Sensory neurons detect changes in their environment, interneurons signal changes to other neurons and motor neurons orchestrate movement, actions and behaviour (Figure 3.2).

- **Grey matter** is dark in colour and made up of neuronal and glial cell bodies and capillaries. This metabolically active tissue uses about 95% of all oxygen delivered to the brain.
- **White matter** is predominantly composed of myelinated nerve fibres that enable rapid conduction of signals between different parts of the nervous system.
- **Synapses** are highly specialised, microscopic connections between neurons that enable the transmission of impulses from one cell to the next by means of neurotransmitter chemicals (Figure 3.4).

Other tissues of the nervous system

Protected by the bones of the **cranium** and the membrane layers known as **meninges**, the brain comprises about 2% of body mass. An extremely rich network of blood vessels nourishes the brain (Chapter 6) and a process known as **autoregulation** tightly regulates blood supply to match the organ's metabolic (energy) demands.

The final component is **cerebrospinal fluid** (CSF), which provides buoyancy, protection and chemical stability (homeostasis) within the environment of the nervous system. CSF is formed by ependymal cells (the choroid plexus) and circulates through the ventricles and spinal cord before being reabsorbed by the arachnoid granulations.

The cerebrum

The largest and most distinctive part of the human brain is responsible for executive functions like conscious experience, thinking, solving problems, learning, decision-making and initiation of movement including speech. The ability to form memories depends on both structural and psychological changes that take place as the cerebrum organises information. Dementia is a progressive disorder, so some functions are retained for longer than others.

Cerebral hemispheres

The two cerebral hemispheres are joined by means of a large bundle of nerve fibres known as the **corpus callosum** that allows information to be passed between them. Each hemisphere controls movement on the opposite side of the body and is made up of four wrinkled lobes with deep folds called **gyri** and creases called **fissures**. The right hemisphere is specialised for recognition of faces and spatial awareness; the left side is specialised for functions such as language, writing and calculation. The **internal capsule** forms a connection between the white matter of the cortical regions by way of the **thalamus**, which serves to relay information to:

- **Frontal lobes**, (Figure 3.3a) which are responsible for higher order processing including personality, judgement, intention and executive functions;
- **Parietal lobes**, which play an important role in bringing together activity from sensory and motor systems, thus enabling sensory perception, spatial awareness and functions such as calculations;
- **Temporal lobes** which include areas that are key for processing sounds and language;
- **Occipital lobes**, which receive information from the eyes and process it to create meaningful, conscious visual images

Basal ganglia

The basal ganglia play an important role in planning of movement (Figure 3.3b). They are composed of clusters of neurons (nuclei) located deep in the cerebrum and include the caudate nucleus, putamen, globus pallidus and substantia nigra.

Limbic structures

In evolutionary terms, this system represents the most primitive part of the cerebral cortex. The limbic cortex (Figure 3.3b) acts as a link between higher cognitive functions like thinking and reason and more instinctive emotional responses such as fear, appetite and anger. The **amygdala** and **cingulate gyrus** are structures that play an important part in emotional responsiveness while the **hippocampus** is crucial to the formation of memories and learning. The limbic system is functionally connected to the **hypothalamus**, which controls basic life processes including circadian rhythms, temperature regulation, appetite, sex drive, thirst and hormone systems.

The brainstem

All information that passes between the spinal cord and cerebrum must pass through the brainstem, which comprises the **midbrain, pons and medulla**. It includes groups of neurons (nuclei) that regulate autonomic activity (Figure 3.2), thus controlling heart rate, blood pressure and breathing. In addition, the **reticular activating system** (RAS) forms a network that plays a key role in modulating levels of consciousness and other responses such as pain.

The cerebellum

The fundamental role of the cerebellum – a very tightly folded layer of grey matter in the hindbrain – is in the fine-tuning of precise, coordinated movement and balance. It is also essential for some kinds of sensorimotor learning, as exemplified by hand–eye coordination, and the ability to analyse visual signals and adjust behaviour accordingly.

4 Progression of dementia

Figure 4.1 **Cognitive reserve helps us to function effectively;** it builds up through intellectual stimulation. Reserve is thought to provide an element of protection that contributes to delaying the changes and clinical symptoms of neuropathology of dementia

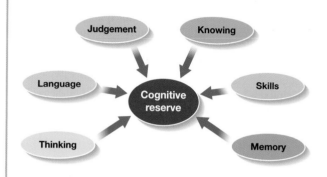

Figure 4.3 **The prevalence of dementia increase with age**

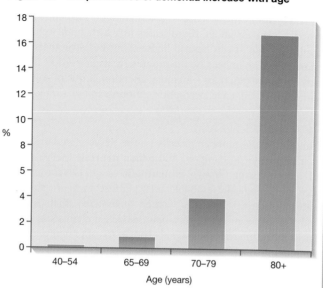

Figure 4.2 **Dendritic spines of neurones are dynamic in shape, volume and size.** They encode changes in the state of individual synapses without affecting the state of other synapses in the same region. This process is key for neuronal plasticity, the basis for memory and learning

Impulses travel towards nerve cell body along a dendrite

Dendrites

Dendritic spines

Nerve cell body

Axon

Nerve impulse travels from cell body along the axon

Axon terminal

Synapse at a dendritic spine

Dendrite of another neuron

Figure 4.4 **Normal brain and brain shrinkage**

(a) **Section of a normal brain and brain of a person affected by Alzheimer's disease** *(right)*

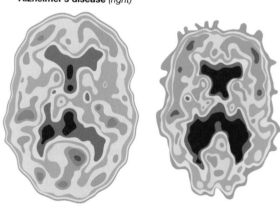

(b) **Normal 80-year-old brain in comparison with that of a person with Alzheimer's disease** *(right)*

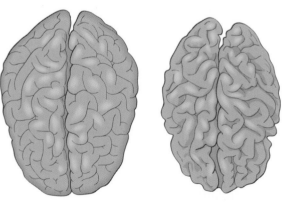

Dementia Care at a Glance, First Edition. Catharine Jenkins, Laura Ginesi and Bernie Keenan. © 2016 by John Wiley & Sons, Ltd. Published 2016 by John Wiley & Sons, Ltd.
Companion website: www.ataglanceseries.com/nursing/dementiacare

The normal ageing brain

Growing older is associated with many physical, biochemical and physiological and psychological changes in the brain. **Plasticity** is the term used to describe the brain's ability to alter structure and networks to function well and perform everyday tasks that we often take for granted. The term **cognitive (mental) reserve** is sometimes used to describe the brain's ability to recruit neural networks in an effective way that enables us to remember, learn new things and live our everyday lives (Figure 4.1). Cognitive reserve seems to build up during a lifetime through intellectual enrichment. However, the extent to which mental stimulation (e.g. puzzles, games, reading) may protect people from aspects of cognitive impairment associated with dementia is still a matter of debate as decline begins at a relatively early age (from the 20s onwards) even in healthy adults.

Advances in neurosciences and imaging technology mean better knowledge of normal age-related brain changes than ever before. At the level of cells, normal cognitive processes and memory ultimately depend on the ability of **neurons** in the brain to fire by creating action potentials and to **communicate** by means of synapses (Chapter 3). With advancing age the density of grey matter and the number of **dendritic spines** on neurons decreases (see Figure 4.2). The changing brain function in normal ageing can be measured in terms of accuracy and speed of information processing, attention, motivation, episodic memory and working memory.

Progression of dementia

The decline in brain function associated with dementia is not the same as normal ageing processes. Dementia is a **syndrome** caused by disease of the brain. Two key **networks**, the hippocampus and the neocortical circuits, appear to be particularly vulnerable to the kinds of **synaptic alteration** that is characteristic of dementia; many biochemical pathways that affect gene expression may be involved. The risk of dementia increases as people get older (Figure 4.3) and it is incurable; the disease cuts lives short, although those affected often die of infections such as pneumonia.

Each person will experience dementia in his or her own way; it is progressive although the rate of decline partly depends on the type of dementia that is affecting the person. Most cases are likely to arise from multiple contributing factors, including the following:

- Degenerative disease of the brain, for example, Alzheimer's disease (Figure 4.4) (Chapter 5), Parkinson's disease or Huntington's disease or vascular dementia (Chapter 6)
- Head injury, for example, stroke related to vascular problems or arrhythmias of heart, single brain trauma or repeated sporting head injury
- Genetic inheritance: for a few families, it may be possible to identify a change to a gene (a mutation) that is responsible in that family
- Infections, for example, Creutzfeldt–Jakob disease and HIV/AIDS
- Exposure to environmental chemicals and contaminants throughout the lifespan and including alcohol or drugs
- Hydrocephalus
- Brain tumours

Those who are affected eventually need help with all aspects of daily living and become increasingly dependent on other people.

There are some broad similarities that include loss of **executive functions** (Figure 4.1) and these **deficits** occur because the brain is becoming progressively damaged by the disease process or small strokes. Age-related sight or hearing loss (Chapter 23) can make things more difficult for people with dementia who may be working hard to make sense of the world around them. There is currently no cure for most types of dementia, but treatments (Chapters 31 and 32), advice and support are available (Chapters 12 and 13).

Signs and symptoms

We may all forget recent conversations or events, but forgetful people can usually still remember other facts related to things they have forgotten. Nevertheless, *decline in short-term memory* is the most apparent early symptom of dementia, but some or all of the following may become increasingly apparent:

- *Changes in mood or behaviour,* for example, mood swings or showing more or less emotion than is usual for the person, or becoming more likely to blame others for mistakes.
- People with dementia may find it *hard to perform familiar tasks to the same standard.* As dementia progresses he or she might start to go wrong when getting dressed, cleaning their teeth or preparing a meal and may get slower at grasping new ideas.
- It is not always easy to spot changes *in personality,* but a person with dementia may become more suspicious, agitated, depressed or irritable than before. He/she may make comments that are hurtful, tell jokes that are offensive or curse and use foul language or display behaviours that are completely out of character.
- Becoming lost in previously familiar places, confusing night and day or forgetting where they are and how they got there are signs of *disorientation to time and place* in the person with dementia.
- People with dementia may be affected by *loss of initiative* so enthusiasm for work, hobbies and everyday activities may disappear and they might spend hours sleeping or sitting.
- Anyone can temporarily forget where they have put things like keys, handbags or wallets, but people with dementia may have *difficulty keeping track of things* including conversations and bills.
- *Problems with language* may mean that a person with dementia substitutes repeats or forgets simple words, all of which may mean it is difficult for family and carers to understand them.

Early diagnosis

Anyone who is experiencing memory problems or is having difficulty when performing everyday tasks should visit their doctor who may be able to exclude other reasons for the difficulties, for example, vitamin deficiencies or thyroid dysfunction.

It is important that people with dementia have an early diagnosis (Chapter 11) and feel supported even if they have been expecting it. People cope better when they understand that changes are the result of the disease process (Chapter 19) rather than a negative aspect of personality. Dementia will increasingly affect judgement and behaviour in ways that are severe enough to affect work, lifelong hobbies and social life, so it is important for those who have been given a diagnosis to find help and support (Chapter 12), put their financial and other affairs in order (Chapter 61) and participate in decisions about their care (Chapter 49) while they still have the capacity to do so.

5 Alzheimer's disease

Figure 5.1 A range of risk factors is associated with Alzheimer's disease

Inherited factors
- Defects in chromosomes 14, 19, 21 for presenilins 1 and 2
- Amyloid precursor protein (APP) and Apolipoprotein E4

Physiological factors
- Older age
- Insulin resistance
- Diabetes
- Adiposity
- Destruction of dendritic spines

Alzheimer's disease

Cellular factors
- Amyloid beta 1-42
- Hyperphosphorylation of tau
- Inflammatory cytokines
- Excitotoxicity
- Oxidative stress

Other factors
- Brain injury
- Sporting head injuries
- Impaired cerebral perfusion
- Higher dietary intake of calories and fat
- Social group
- Ethnicity

Figure 5.2 Alzheimer's disease – neuropathological hallmarks:

(a) Neurofibrillary tangles

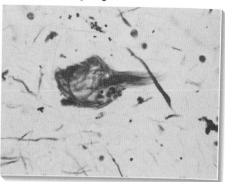

(b) Neuritic plaques

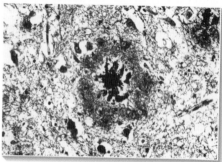

Source: *Reproduced with permission of Lionel Ginsberg*

Figure 5.3 All proteins begin as a string of amino acids (a peptide) which folds into a three-dimensional shape that allows it to perform useful functions within our cells. Manifestation of Alzheimer's pathology is characterised by deposits of amyloid-beta (Aβ), an insoluble, mis-folded peptide. All the molecular complexes involved in the enzyme cascade process leading to Aβ are located in the membrane of neurons

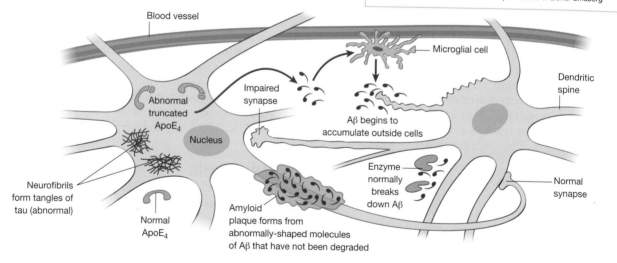

Figure 5.4 The architectural framework of all human cells depends on the cytoskeleton which consists of protein microfilaments and microtubules. In Alzheimer's disease, the abnormal strands of tau form tangles leading to decreased capacity for dendritic spine formation

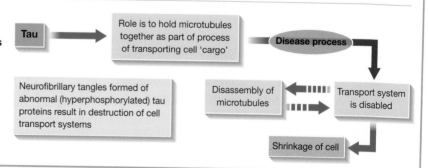

Dementia Care at a Glance, First Edition. Catharine Jenkins, Laura Ginesi and Bernie Keenan. © 2016 by John Wiley & Sons, Ltd. Published 2016 by John Wiley & Sons, Ltd.
Companion website: www.ataglanceseries.com/nursing/dementiacare

Overview

Alzheimer's disease (AD), the most common form of dementia, accounts for 60–70% of all dementias. The progressive nature of AD causes stress for the affected person and their loved ones, carers and families. A major barrier to effective treatments is an incomplete understanding of the mechanism of development of the disease.

Old age is the strongest risk factor, but identification of the populations at greatest risk of AD is confounded by differences/disparities in the burden of risk factors (see Figure 5.1). For example, development of AD is accelerated in patients with diabetes or those who have received head injuries in sports like boxing or rugby. Other characteristics associated with a higher risk of AD include lower socioeconomic status, lower level of education and minority ethnicity.

Estimates of the number of people affected vary, but generally it is thought that one in 14 people over 65 years of age and one in six over 80 years of age have AD or another neurodegenerative disease associated with disability and a need for professional care.

AD is not a normal part of ageing

Normal neurotransmission is crucial for the brain to function well and the progressive memory loss and behavioural change of AD is caused by disruption of crucial communications within the brain (see Figure 4.2).

Alois Alzheimer, a psychiatrist and neuropathologist, was the first person to describe the **microscopic** changes known as **neuritic plaques** and **neurofibrillary tangles** (see Figure 5.2) in the brain of a person with dementia. Post-mortem examination reveals that the brains of people who have been affected by the disease that bears his name are distinctive and changed from normal; the cerebral cortex shrinks (atrophies) and the amount of brain tissue is reduced. Some parts of the brain diminish progressively, others seem completely unaffected across the lifespan. For example, pyramidal cells in the prefrontal association cortex are affected early and severely while cells in sensory areas, including the visual cortex, are usually changed very little, even in late-stage disease. The precise mechanism in AD remains controversial, but it is clear that extensive degeneration of interconnections between neurons (synapses) through cell death occurs over a long period. Ultimately, these molecular events and cellular changes have an impact on cognitive abilities required for everyday living (see Chapter 4).

Amyloid cascade hypothesis

The leading pathophysiological explanation for AD is based on a theory that an abnormal form of a protein called **amyloid** accumulates to form hallmark **senile plaques** that are a defining feature of the disease. In particular, **amyloid-beta** (Aβ) fragments (Figure 5.3) precipitate and form abnormal, insoluble clumps (aggregates) in the **extracellular space** around neurons (Figure 5.2b). **Posterior cortical atrophy (PCA)** is a rare and atypical presentation of AD in which the amyloid load is similar but the early stages are characterised by visual disturbances.

Hyperphosphorylation of tau

Flame-shaped **neurofibrillary tangles** (NFTs), another characteristic of AD, are deposits of a different abnormal protein inside neurons (Figure 5.2a). Normally, the physiological role of **tau** is to help maintain the stability of **microtubules**, which are part of the architectural framework (**cytoskeleton**) that is crucial for many cell functions including division, motility, flexibility and differentiation. If the cytoskeleton breaks down, then cells cannot function.

In AD, a biochemical process called **hyperphosphorylation of tau** selectively affects pyramidal neurons, which are highly branched cells located in the cerebral cortex, the hippocampus and the amygdala (part of the limbic cortex) (see Chapter 3). The changes seem to induce generalised collapse of microtubules, leading to disconnection between the many other neurons they connect with and eventual memory loss (see Figure 5.4). AD is, therefore, one of the best-known examples of a group of diseases known as **tauopathies.**

Multiple neurotoxic pathways

The plaques and tangles have long been considered toxic to the brain, but smaller, soluble forms of Aβ may be causing neuronal injury and contribute to cell death through:

- **Neuroinflammation:** cells from the immune system (*microglia*) have been found in amyloid plaques, suggesting that damage to the brain associated with AD could derive from an autoimmune response.
- **Excitotoxicity:** the neurotransmitter *glutamate* is thought to be particularly involved in primary perception and cognition. Aβ may trigger a spreading cascade of over-activation of glutamatergic circuits that induces further damage to neurons and results in cognitive aspects of the disorder (Chapter 19).
- **Mitochondrial dysfunction:** aerobic energy production by cells is dependent on these tiny dynamic organelles. Excitotoxicity may render them incapable of performing their crucial functions within neurons as a result of severe swelling.
- **oxidative stress:** an imbalance between production of **reactive oxygen species** (ROS), sometimes called free radicals, and an inability of cells to defend against their effects damages nucleic acids, proteins and lipids and cell structures such as mitochondria.

Genetic risk factors for AD

Genetic (non-modifiable) factors are implicated in fewer than 5% of all cases of AD. Nevertheless, in some families, there seems to be a clear pattern of inheritance that includes changes in the DNA sequences (**mutations**) of genes that code for **amyloid precursor protein** (APP) and **presenilin(s)** (see Figure 5.3). Defects in **apolipoprotein E4** (ApoE4), which binds beta-amyloid, are associated with a higher risk of early age of onset because other forms of ApoE appear to be protective.

Other factors

The human brain is very vulnerable to disruptions in **glucose supply** and **oxygen delivery** (Chapter 6) because its function is completely dependent on aerobic respiration. Indeed, glucose metabolism in the brain is reduced in patients with mild cognitive impairment (MCI) and utilisation is severely **impaired** in some regions in the early stages of AD and following stroke or other acquired brain injury (Figure 5.1).

There is a growing body of evidence to suggest that the physiological basis for both **type 2 diabetes mellitus** (T2DM) and AD is related to chronic, systemic impairment in glucose metabolism and utilisation known as **insulin resistance** (Chapter 10). However, it is difficult to determine whether poor cerebral blood flow and insulin resistance are consequences of AD or a primary cause. Many AD patients have signs of atherosclerosis (Chapter 6), while neuronal insulin resistance could be a consequence of toxicity of Aβ.

6 Vascular dementia

Figure 6.1 Infarcts and occlusion can arise within the cerebral circulation because of thrombosis, embolism, microbleeds or lacunar disease

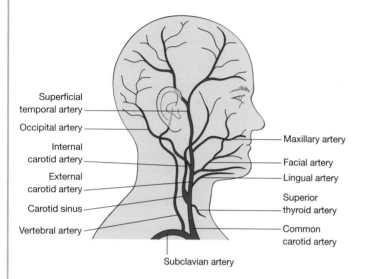

(a) **Blood supply of the head and neck**

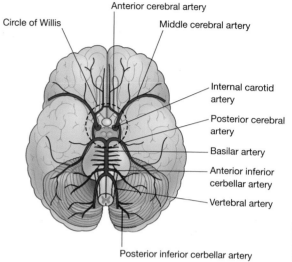

(b) **Blood supply of the brain**

Vascular diseases and conditions associated with cognitive impairments and dementia

Range of pathophysiology develops because of infarcts (ischaemia) in the brain

Vascular dementias

Mixed dementia

Alzheimer's disease and VaD co-exist in 50% of patients

Mild cognitive impairment

Does not meet formal criteria for dementia

Table 6.1 Adequate cerebral blood flow is essential for normal function.
Pressures within the arterial system must be enough to supply blood to the head and cranial cavity

Parameter	Normal range	Additional information
Cerebral blood flow (CBF)	45–60 cm³/100 g of tissue/min	Perfusion is regulated by metabolic demands within the cranium, blood gases, pH, local vasodilators and neural input. If CBF falls to less than 18–20 cm³/100 g/min, homeostasis is disturbed, often irreversibly
Intracranial pressure (ICP)	10–15 mmHg	The 3 components that contribute to ICP are volume of brain tissue, volume of blood within the cranium and volume of cerebrospinal fluid (CSF)
Cerebral perfusion pressure (CPP)	70–100 mmHg	This is the pressure required to deliver blood to the brain and cranial vault. It is the mean arterial blood pressure (MAP) minus intracranial pressure (ICP), i.e. CPP = MAP − ICP
Autoregulatory range	50–150 mmHg	Myogenic, neurogenic and metabolic factors contribute to ways in which cerebral blood vessels are able to constrict or dilate to regulate perfusion (flow) to the brain. If mean arterial pressure (MAP) is below 50 mmHg, there is not enough force to deliver blood to the brain; if it exceeds 150 mmHg, cerebral vessels are damaged and the integrity of the blood–brain barrier is compromised

Dementia Care at a Glance, First Edition. Catharine Jenkins, Laura Ginesi and Bernie Keenan. © 2016 by John Wiley & Sons, Ltd. Published 2016 by John Wiley & Sons, Ltd.
Companion website: www.ataglanceseries.com/nursing/dementiacare

Vascular dementia

Vascular dementia (VaD) occurs because blood supply to parts of the cortex and sub-cortex is interrupted (see Figure 6.1). It affects 10–15% of all people with dementia and used to be known as multi-infarct dementia. VaD is the second most common form of dementia, the symptoms of VaD develop in ways that are individual to the patient because they are determined by the location of the infarct (area of interrupted supply). The frontal lobes of the cerebral hemispheres are particularly vulnerable due to their relative size.

People who have this form of dementia do not necessarily present with memory dysfunction. VaD often manifests through alterations in behaviour and/or difficulties with executive functions such as thinking, planning, weighing up long-term consequences, problem-solving and/or organisation. Loss of these skills and abilities can have devastating consequences on a person's ability to perform complex yet everyday tasks like choosing and preparing a meal. People with VaD often have more insight into their condition. They can be prone to depression and labile, or swiftly changing, moods.

In at least 50% of VaD patients, mixed pathology with Alzheimer's disease (AD) is apparent, and both diseases have some commonality in risk factors, for example, hypertension, abdominal obesity, insulin resistance, diabetes mellitus, smoking, dyslipidaemia and high levels of homocysteine (Chapter 10).

The cerebral circulation

The brain has a very high demand for aerobic production of adenosine triphosphate (ATP) compared with other organs, so constant supply of oxygen and nutrients is critical for function. As a result, 15–20% of cardiac output is delivered to brain tissue through a network of vessels that is estimated to be 400 miles long and has some special properties.

- The capillaries of the brain are supplied with blood by means of two arterial systems. The internal carotids and basilar arteries are connected via the circle of Willis (see Figure 6.1), an anatomical mechanism that reduces haemodynamic stress and ensures that brain tissue receives compensatory (collateral) blood supply when there is a blockage.
- Cerebral autoregulation is the ability of the brain to maintain adequate blood flow across a wide range of arterial pressures (see Table 6.1) through processes that are regulated by a combination of myogenic properties of vascular smooth muscle and metabolic factors including carbon dioxide, nitric oxide and potassium (K^+). Significant injury follows disruption of autoregulatory processes, for example as a consequence of severe hypertension.

The function of neurons, oligodendrocytes, astrocytes and microglia (Chapter 3) are all extremely sensitive to oxygen deprivation (hypoxia); major vascular events may be preceded by periods of chronic hypoxia if cerebral blood flow (CBF) falls below 18–20 cm^3/100 g/min. To an extent, collateral networks including the Circle of Willis allow blood to pass between systems for redistribution and drainage when conduits fail, but a reduction in CBF that is characteristic of VaD starts early; if it is less than 8–10 cm^3/100 g/min, neuronal tissue dies (infarction).

Impaired perfusion of cerebral vessels ('brain attack')

The course of VaD is more gradual than AD but may also be abrupt or stepwise because VaD is caused by multiple (often small) strokes. Ischaemia, which can be partial or complete, occurs when an artery or arteriole becomes narrow or obstructed, allowing less blood to flow through it. As a result, the microenvironment of cells in the brain may change, leading to adaptive processes that contribute to cellular malfunction and cell death (necrosis). Magnetic resonance imaging (MRI) is often used in people who have cognitive impairment to evaluate changes to vessels in the brain as evidence of VaD.

Atherosclerosis of cerebral arteries

Arteries become clogged with fatty material (cholesterol, fibrous and connective tissue) that is deposited in and under the lining of arteries. The immune system responds with inflammatory processes leading to formation of blood clots (thrombi) that can block the vessel completely. Sometimes an artery or arteriole becomes blocked with material that originated elsewhere in the body and moved through the circulatory system until it became trapped (embolism). Clots can also form because of heart valve abnormalities and arrhythmias, for example, atrial fibrillation. The subsequent level of impairment of the person's cognitive function will depend on where the blockage occurred and resultant areas of ischaemia. A large embolus may cause stroke or transient ischaemic attack (TIA), whereas the cumulative effect of many small, asymptomatic emboli causes progressive damage over a significantly longer period.

Haemorrhagic stroke

If cerebral blood vessels rupture, for example, from an aneurysm, blood enters the brain substance or the subarachnoid space. The bleed may manifest as a severe headache of sudden origin (thunderclap). As with other forms of cerebrovascular disease, the pattern of deficits depends on the location and size of the lesion.

Cerebral amyloid angiopathy

This condition occurs when the protein amyloid is deposited in the walls of blood vessels, causing them to crack and leak. However, it is important to note that the term amyloid describes a range of proteins (not necessarily related to each other) and the amyloid in cerebral amyloid angiopathy is not the same as amyloid in AD.

Cerebral small vessel disease

Age-related alterations in the structure of small arterioles are characteristic of this disease, sometimes known as subcortical ischaemic VaD (SIVD), and found in 60–70% of people who have VaD. Other names are leucoaraiosis or vascular leucoencephalopathy and the disease particularly affects subcortical structures including basal ganglia, deep white matter in thalamus and cerebellum and the pons (Chapter 3). Long, penetrating end arterioles travel for a long distance from the surface and base of the brain to supply the deep white matter; the lumen becomes stenosed and the abnormal areas (white matter lesions) can be viewed by computed tomography (CT) scan or MRI. Lacunar infarcts are changes in the white matter that typically involve ischaemia, demyelination, astrogliosis and axon loss; they are thought to cause dementia by disrupting and disconnecting pathways between cortical and subcortical centres.

7 Less common forms of dementia

Figure 7.1 Events at a synapse where neurotransmitter is released on demand by exocytosis

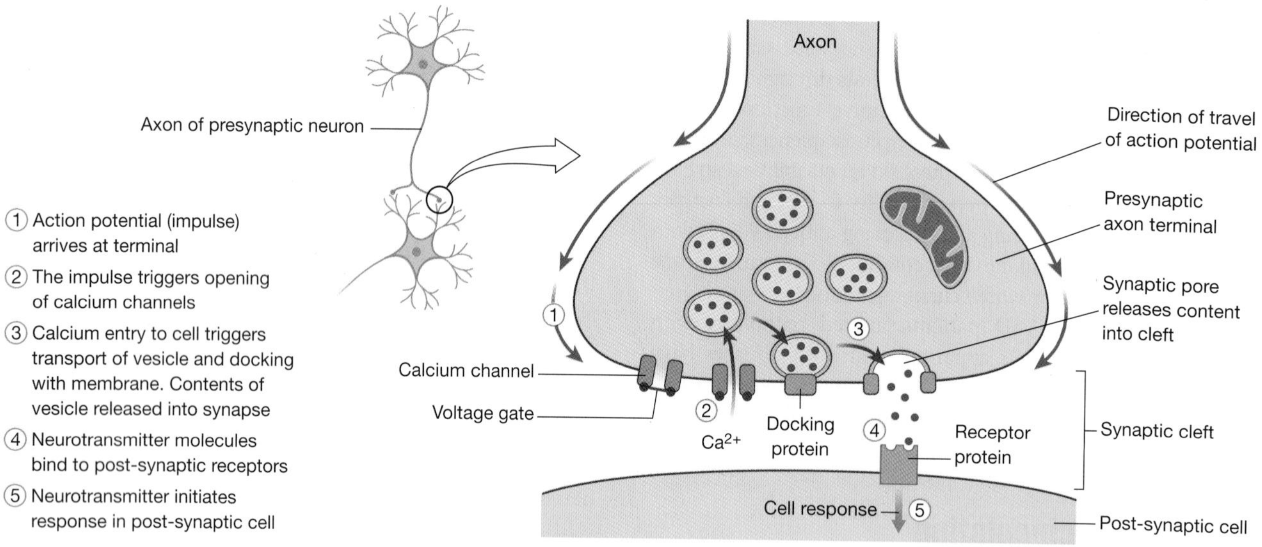

① Action potential (impulse) arrives at terminal

② The impulse triggers opening of calcium channels

③ Calcium entry to cell triggers transport of vesicle and docking with membrane. Contents of vesicle released into synapse

④ Neurotransmitter molecules bind to post-synaptic receptors

⑤ Neurotransmitter initiates response in post-synaptic cell

Table 7.1 Characteristics of some important types of dementia

Condition	Alzheimer's disease	Dementia with Lewy bodies	Fronto-temporal dementia (Pick's disease)	Creutzveldt-Jacob dementia	Posterior cortical atrophy	HIV dementia complex
Cellular characteristics	Neuritic plaques containing beta amyloid	Amyloid plaques	Some neurons have Pick bodies; cells may swell (ballooning) and die; gliosis (nerve tissue scarring) and vacuolation create 'holes' in the outer layer of brain	Appearance of abnormal prion proteins leading to neuronal loss	High amyloid-β load in the occipital cortex	Virus infects cells that normally nurture support neurons; the infected cells activate brain-specific immune cells that instruct neurons to undergo cell death (apoptosis)
	Neurofibrillary tangles of abnormal tau	Lewy bodies deposits of alpha-synuclein	Abnormal tau in Pick bodies; some inclusions contain abnormal DNA-binding TDP-43; or fused in sarcoma (FUS) protein	Aggregates of abnormal prion proteins	CSF markers and other pathophysiology tend to indicate atypical Alzheimer's disease	The infected support cells secrete neurotoxic substances; this behavior is harmful for neurons leading to their destruction
Part of the brain that is affected	Parietal, temporal and parieto-occipital cortex	Fronto-temporal regions of cortex	Fronto-temporal regions of cortex	Brain tissue becomes filled with microscopic holes	Predominantly regions of the parieto-occipital cortex; temporal regions are relatively spared	Subcortical; basal ganglia
Other aspects	Deficits in acetylcholine	Deficits in acetylcholine and dopamine	Genetic component in 10–20% of cases of FTD	Brain tissue resembles a sponge hence the term spongiform encephalopathy	Glucose hypo-metabolism	Also known as HIV-associated dementia (HAD) and HIV encephalopathy (HIE)
Manifestations	Memory loss, impaired learning, progressive behaviour change	Delirium, executive functions, delusions, depression, visual hallucinations, REM sleep disorder,	Poor judgement; impaired speech and language; compulsive behaviours; lack of empathy; decline in social and personal contact; euphoria, depression, apathy; decline in personal hygiene	Sporadic CJD makes up the majority of cases; the inherited form is rare. The infective agent for bovine spongiform encephalopathy (BSE) in cows is believed to be the same responsible for new variant CJD (nvCJD) in humans	Insidious onset of visual disturbances, followed by impairment of visuospatial skills. Episodic memory and insight are relatively spared	Mental slowing, poor concentration, apathy altered posture and gait similar to those observed in advanced Parkinson's disease
Movement-related disorders	Rare	Parkinsonism within a year of onset	Some subtypes: tremor and rigidity, muscle weakness/spasm, poor coordination and difficulty in swallowing	Lack of coordination (e.g. changes in gait stumbling and falling); muscle twitching, seizures or stiffness; impaired speech	Progression includes poor hand-eye coordination (ataxia), inability to write or recognise own fingers	Slowness in execution of movements (bradykinesia), clumsiness, poor balance

Dementia Care at a Glance, First Edition. Catharine Jenkins, Laura Ginesi and Bernie Keenan. © 2016 by John Wiley & Sons, Ltd. Published 2016 by John Wiley & Sons, Ltd.
Companion website: www.ataglanceseries.com/nursing/dementiacare

In a healthy brain, the number of cells and speed of functioning may decline in adulthood, but the organ continues to form new connections and memories (plasticity). However, when connections are lost through inflammation, disease or injury, neurons eventually die and dementia may result (Table 7.1). Here we describe some of the less common forms of dementia, although this is not an exhaustive list.

Dementia with Lewy bodies

In people who have dementia with Lewy bodies (DLB), fluctuations in level of alertness/drowsiness and sleep disorders may occur over periods ranging from a few hours to days or weeks. The affected person may have recurrent, vivid and detailed visual hallucinations. Other manifestations of DLB include dysfunction of the autonomic nervous system. This form of dementia is characterised by the formation of inclusion bodies within the cytoplasm of neurons. These structures are different from the neuritic plaques and neurofibrillary tangles characteristic of Alzheimer's disease (AD) (Chapter 5). Loss of cholinergic (acetylcholine-producing) neurons is thought to be responsible for the decline in cognitive function while death of dopaminergic (dopamine-producing) neurons affects the initiation and cessation of voluntary and involuntary movements (parkinsonism) leading to stiffness and balance problems.

Alpha-synuclein (aSyn), a small protein of 140 amino acids, may be dysfunctional in DLB, Parkinson's disease (PD) and other degenerative conditions. Although the physiological role of α-synuclein within cells is not well understood, it is a protein for maintaining the supply of synaptic vesicles, which are essential for communication between neurons (Figure 7.1). Outside the cell, aSyn may modulate the neuro-inflammation and glial cell function.

The impact of DLB on the affected person is associated with the location of the Lewy body aggregates within the brain and the extent of any Alzheimer's pathology that may also co-occur. Indeed, in the early stages, DLB may be confused with AD and vascular dementia (VaD), but despite this difficulty, it is important that DLB is promptly diagnosed because people with DLB are hypersensitive to some neuroleptic drugs and because appropriate treatment can improve life for the affected person and his/her caregivers.' Could we divide it so it is like this: 'Indeed, in the early stages, DLB may be confused with AD and vascular dementia (VaD). However, despite this difficulty, it is important that DLB is promptly diagnosed because people with DLB are hypersensitive to some neuroleptic drugs and because appropriate treatment can improve life for the affected person and his/her caregivers.

Frontotemporal dementia including Pick's disease

A slow process of shrinkage (atrophy) of the frontal lobes and temporal lobes of the brain is the common feature of a relatively rare group of conditions that usually appear when someone is in their mid-40s to early 60s. Frontotemporal dementia (FTD) causes a steady, irreversible deterioration of an individual's ability to think and function over a period of years. Because the regions of the brain that are key for speech and language as well as personality are affected, people with FTD may make rude, inappropriate remarks or do things that are dangerous. Each subtype produces different symptoms, but all the types eventually leave the person completely dependent on caregivers.

In some patients, the affected parts of the brain contain cells with Pick bodies (microscopic accumulations of abnormal tau) and this is why FTD used to be known as Pick's disease. However, other accumulations in FTD involve the protein TDP-43, so the term Pick's disease is no longer used very often.

Caregivers sometimes report that they feel embarrassed or frustrated. They often find the sudden verbal outbursts, impulsive behaviours and 'food fads' are out of character for the affected person, so it is important to remember that there is a physical cause and that the person has little ability to control or have insight into their behaviour. Nevertheless, remembering how the person was before he/she was affected by FTD is extremely distressing for loved ones; seeking support and taking time for themselves can help family members and caregivers to cope.

Korsakoff's syndrome

A chronic deficiency of thiamine (vitamin B_{12}) contributes to the neuronal loss, micro-haemorrhages and glial (supporting) cells that are associated with this preventable form of dementia. Episodic memory formation is severely impaired (anterograde amnesia) in patients with Korsakoff's syndrome (also known as Korsakoff's psychosis, alcohol related dementia or amnesic-confabulatory syndrome) while memory for perceptual and motor skills remains intact. The dementia arises because of deranged metabolic processes in parts of the brain and limbic cortex that are important for processing of memory, words and mood. In Western nations, the most common causes of such a deficiency are alcoholism, eating disorders and chemotherapy, but people with Korsakoff's syndrome may be capable of new learning, particularly if they live in a calm, supportive and well-structured environment.

Creutzfeldt–Jakob disease

This is a rare form of degenerative disease that causes relatively rapid deterioration. In the early stages, the person may have failing memory, changes in behaviour and problems with muscular coordination and may experience visual disturbance. Involuntary jerky movements (myoclonus) often develop and people eventually lose the ability to move and speak, eventually entering a coma. The prognosis is poor and 90% of affected individuals die within a year. Several variants of Creutzfeldt–Jakob disease (CJD) have been identified, each of which differs in its course. The disease belongs to a group of transmissible spongiform encephalopathies (TSEs), which are caused by prion proteins. Normally these are harmless proteins found in body cells, but an infectious form of prions, which have characteristics different from bacteria, viruses or other infectious agents, seem to form spontaneously and trigger a chain reaction that alters proteins in other cells.

Huntington's disease

Huntington's disease is an inherited (autosomal dominant) degenerative disease of movement with behavioural disturbance and progressive dementia that usually begins during mid-life.

Mixed dementia

Mixed dementia refers to a combination of AD, vascular ischaemia and other dementia disorders. It is evident from post-mortems that a large proportion of people have signs of AD and VaD. Nevertheless, making the distinction between these diseases can be difficult because of the interactions between their effects and impact on the individual; the combination of two forms of dementia may have greater impact than either on its own.

8 Younger people with dementia

Table 8.1 Ways in which living with a person with dementia may affect children and teenagers

Parent's (or person with dementia's) perspective	Child or teen's perspective on the situation	Consequence for child or teen	Feelings related to being told what is happening
Desire to protect child or teen from difficult/confusing situation	Child or teen is aware of tension and troubled atmosphere	Worries related to belief that the person's behaviour is their fault	News of the illness may be distressing
Avoiding telling children or teenagers the facts about dementia	Can be upsetting to find the truth out at a later stage	May not trust people who are close to them	Relief that the person's behaviour is part of an illness rather than being directed at them
Unpleasant task to explain dementia	Grief and sadness at what is happening to someone they love	Anxiety about an uncertain future for their loved one	Learning to manage painful emotions and difficult situations
Lack of insight into changing behaviour	Boredom when hearing the same thing over and over again	Embarrassment about unusual behaviour in front of others	Guilt for experiencing deep feelings and loss
Inability to communicate well with the child or teen	Confusion about role reversal and being responsible for their parent	May feel that parents have less time for them; isolation, anger or rejection	Sense of powerlessness because of inability to change the situation or help their loved one get better
Talking about the impact of dementia on the family	May be afraid to talk to adults because they are already under strain	Inability to explain the situation to school friends and others	Reassurance that the illness is the problem not their loved one

Table 8.2 Impact of a parent with dementia on a child or teenager

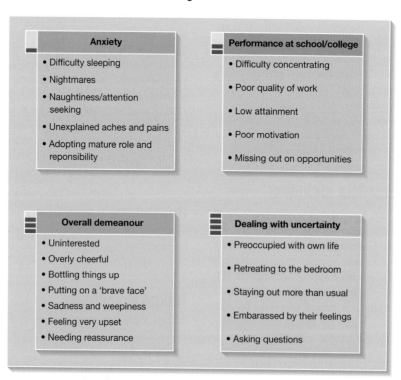

Dementia Care at a Glance, First Edition. Catharine Jenkins, Laura Ginesi and Bernie Keenan. © 2016 by John Wiley & Sons, Ltd. Published 2016 by John Wiley & Sons, Ltd.
Companion website: www.ataglanceseries.com/nursing/dementiacare

Context and statistics

Dementia is generally associated with old age, but a significant number (~17,000 in the United Kingdom) of younger people, aged between 30 and 65 years, are living with dementia. Rarer forms of dementia tend to be associated with younger age groups, and the initial signs may not be associated with dementia, but gradually symptoms become similar to those experienced by older people. The context of people's life stages makes early-onset dementia (EOD) particularly challenging for people of working age and their families, which may include their children. In addition, because dementia is not expected in younger people, assessment, diagnosis, support and services can be difficult to access.

Causation

Dementia in younger people (below the age of 65 years) may be caused by Alzheimer's disease (Chapter 5) or vascular disease (Chapter 6). However, larger numbers of younger people are affected by less common causes such as prefrontal dementia, rare inherited conditions, prion disease (e.g. Creutzfeldt–Jakob disease), metabolic disorders, head injury, alcohol-related dementia or dementia caused by conditions such as Parkinson's disease or Huntington's disease (Chapter 7). People with learning disabilities are particularly vulnerable to EOD; for example, there is an association between Down's syndrome and Alzheimer's disease (Chapter 9).

Recognition and assessment

Low mood, irritability, poor concentration, poor work performance and personality changes may be the first indications of problems. Although they are unlikely to be interpreted as signs of dementia, the changes may alienate colleagues, partners and friends. Early symptoms vary, depending on the cause, and may include language problems (semantic dementia) difficulties with visual recognition (posterior cortical atrophy) or uncharacteristic self-centredness or disinhibition (frontotemporal dementia). Memory problems are often not the first problems to be noticed in younger people with dementia.

The wide range of initial difficulties together with the rareness of the conditions means there is a risk of misdiagnosis and the correct diagnosis of dementia can take a long time. People with EOD are sometimes initially diagnosed with other mental health problems such as depression, anxiety or schizophrenia. Specialist assessment is essential to ensure potentially treatable causes are ruled out and to enable the affected person and his or her family to gain access to treatment and support. Sometimes newly diagnosed people feel suicidal. Pre-diagnostic counselling is part of the process. The person should be asked whether they wish to know their diagnosis and consent to the tests. Assessment includes a thorough physical examination, blood tests, specialist scans (e.g. MRI), cognitive tests and conversations with the person and someone who knows them well, to explore the history of the problem.

Life-stage and family issues

Younger people with dementia confront difficulties related to work, family and financial responsibilities. The affected person may have roles and responsibilities including paying a mortgage, supporting a partner and bringing up children. The impact on family life (Table 8.1) and financial planning can be overwhelming. People with EOD may also have older parents or other relatives who need support and their own spouse/partner may be in work.

In the early stages, family members may not understand the reasons for behavioural changes and may misinterpret them in ways that damage relationships, for example children may perceive their parent as uninterested or irritable (Table 8.2) while a spouse/partner may wonder whether the person they love is having a breakdown or an affair. For these reasons, carers of younger people with dementia experience significantly higher levels of stress than those of older people with dementia.

Care and interventions

The pathway to sources of support or services is often unclear. Younger people with dementia are likely to be physically active and otherwise healthy. They may take driving, sporting activity and sexual relationships for granted, while family members, friends and professionals may have concerns about risks, particularly if the person does not have insight into their difficulties. Counselling and support, plus advice about finances, workplace issues and benefits are essential for enabling decision-making while the person has the capacity to contribute. Family therapy can assist in relatives adapting emotionally and practically to the current and future situation. A parent's condition should be explained sensitively to children, using language they are able to understand.

Specialised care for younger people with dementia is not available in all areas and services provided for older people are not suitable because activities and expectations are age-related. Younger people living with dementia benefit from age-appropriate interventions that recognise their norms and provide opportunities to exercise, to mix socially and offer mutual support. Individualised care and respite is best carried out in a familiar home environment, by trained nurses and nursing assistants with specialised communication skills, who have got to know the person well.

Later stages and specialist care

Younger people with dementia may remain physically strong while experiencing serious problems in their abilities to communicate, understand others and to manage basic activities such as washing, dressing, eating and using the toilet. When frustrated they may become distressed or aggressive towards others. If professional care is needed, then this should be in a specialised environment where staff are trained to cope with the specific needs of younger people with dementia. There should be plenty of opportunities to exercise outdoors, to take part in activities, and contribute to day-to-day household business like cooking. Outings and special events raise morale. Family members should be included and feel they are an on-going part of the person's life.

9 People with learning disabilities and dementia

Figure 9.1 Down's syndrome is a genetic condition caused by an extra chromosome

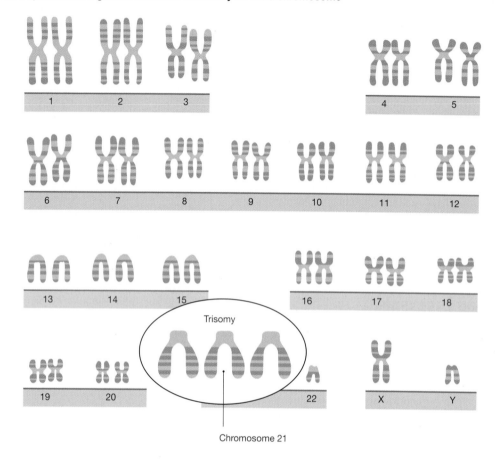

Table 9.1 Assessment, interventions and adaptations

Area for assessment	Example of change	Potential interventions and adaptations
Mood	Feeling sad, low in mood or uncharacteristically irritable or frustrated Lability of mood – the person's mood changes rapidly	Arrange an assessment of mood, as anti-depressants could be helpful. Reassure the person using verbal and non-verbal communication. Include him or her and make opportunities for enjoyable activities and the company of friends and family. Remain calm, listen to distress and validate emotions, then lead into an activity which will occupy and distract
Memory	The person may forget what they have said or done recently. They may not take in information that others tell them. Their vocabulary will diminish, both expressively and receptively, making communication more difficult. They may forget the way around or how to do tasks which keep them independent	Respond to repetition as if it is the first time – do not point out mistakes. Use non-verbal communication to reinforce spoken language. Use the language that the person learnt first, as far as possible. Combine languages to see which is the most effective, for example Makaton with first language. Provide an environment with plenty of cues, such as signs and labels. Ensure the person has their glasses and hearing aid if they need them
Behaviour	The person may repeat activities or 'get stuck' on one part of a task. Risks might arise with managing money, cooking, bathing or crossing the road. They may react in a disinhibited way and forget social skills. They might feel vulnerable and show the need for protection from others by following loved ones around, or becoming distressed if they do not know where they are	Prompt as necessary to aid the person, aim to maintain independence and self-esteem. Interpret the meaning of the behaviour and aim to meet any indicated unmet need. Reassure the person and offer help when needed. Listen and aim to help the person feel understood and valued

Dementia Care at a Glance, First Edition. Catharine Jenkins, Laura Ginesi and Bernie Keenan. © 2016 by John Wiley & Sons, Ltd. Published 2016 by John Wiley & Sons, Ltd.
Companion website: www.ataglanceseries.com/nursing/dementiacare

Old age and learning or intellectual disability

People with learning or intellectual disabilities are living longer, but they experience age-related problems at earlier chronological ages than others. As part of this premature ageing, they are more likely to have physical health problems such as circulatory and mobility difficulties. They also have much higher risk of developing dementia, with almost all people over 40 years of age with Down's syndrome having the senile plaques and neurofibrillary tangles associated with dementia (Prasher, 2005). People with Down's syndrome then tend to go on to develop dementia in their 40s and 50s. However, not all people with intellectual disabilities other than Down's syndrome, or Down's syndrome itself, develop dementia.

Genetic factors

The most common intellectual disability is Down's syndrome, which is caused by an extra copy of chromosome 21 (Figure 9.1). Genes located on this chromosome are responsible for governing the behaviour of amyloid beta proteins and tau, which lead to the plaques and tangles believed to cause Alzheimer's disease. The extra copy of the gene means increased risk of dementia for people with Down's syndrome.

Recognition

It is more difficult to recognise signs of dementia in people who also have learning disabilities. Changes may be very subtle and other people may not notice or, in a process known as 'diagnostic overshadowing', may believe any difficulties are caused by the learning disability itself. People with learning disabilities often have complex health and social needs so in addition it is difficult to ascertain the causes and inter-relationships between these issues. Within this complicated picture, the person may also be cared for by people who have not known them for long enough to be able to note changes and who in addition may not be trained in the signs to observe.

The person with learning disabilities may not know how to explain the changes they are experiencing through verbal communication and could express frustration in other ways. Low mood is also often associated with development of dementia, but this sign could be understood by other people to be caused by losses such as bereavement of family members or friends. If the person has always had limited abilities to self-care, then gradual deterioration may not be noticed.

Poor physical health, epileptic seizures, mobility problems and pain may all contribute to the complex picture. The benefit of recognition is that it should lead to assessment, which in turn can lead to the provision of more suitable support, treatment and care. A baseline of the person's abilities and strengths, together with any care needs, made before the age of 40 years, is helpful for future reference, as more accurate comparisons can be made. Areas to note changes in include memory, mood and behaviour (Table 9.1).

Family, friends and carer issues

Dementia causes similar problems for people with learning difficulties as it does for the general population, but the context of the difficulties mean the problems can have a more serious impact, earlier in the person's life and when their support network may also be weaker. Parents who are carers will be getting older and are likely to express concerns about their own ability to cope and about what would happen to their adult child should they die. They may also wonder whether the person would be better in shared accommodation with others with learning disabilities or whether to plan for extra support in the home environment or for specialised care, for example, in a nursing home. Changing care needs may lead to relocation, but this sometimes exacerbates the problems associated with dementia. Pathways to care may not be clear and family members may be concerned about media or other reports of inadequate or even harmful care environments. The friendship group of the person with learning disabilities will gradually reduce as they develop illnesses and may die earlier. It is difficult to explain the changes associated with dementia, and friends may become upset by uncharacteristic behaviour.

Problems associated with dementia

In common with other people with dementia, people with learning difficulties will develop problems with:

- language, for example using nouns. They may forget what they have said and repeat themselves.
- orientating themselves even in familiar places.
- mixing up night and day and having a disturbed sleep pattern.
- recognising people, particularly those they do not see frequently.
- 'sequencing' (do things in the right order) tasks – for example making tea, meaning they become less independent, which can be frustrating for them and not easily understood by others.
- becoming disinhibited and responding in ways that are difficult to cope with, for example, in sexual or aggressive behaviour, particularly if they feel frightened, annoyed or embarrassed.
- continence, because they do not recognise the need to use the toilet or have forgotten where it is.
- eating more or less than previously, having either forgotten to eat or that they have already eaten, and so lose or gain weight.

Approaches to care

The person with learning disabilities and dementia will inevitably need more support as the condition progresses. It is important to explain what is happening early in the condition, using language the person can relate to, so that they can express their wishes and make decisions in advance. Care should be provided in a safe, ideally familiar environment, which provides opportunities for maximising independence and fun. Practical issues such as hearing, eyesight and pain management, together with personal requirements for well-being, including spirituality issues, will need to be incorporated into care. The ideal approach is person-centred, in which carers know the person and their history well; they should take time to communicate sensitively while aiming to problem solve if difficulties arise. Professional learning disability carers will need training in dementia care so as to add this specific expertise to the wide range of skills needed to address complex care needs.

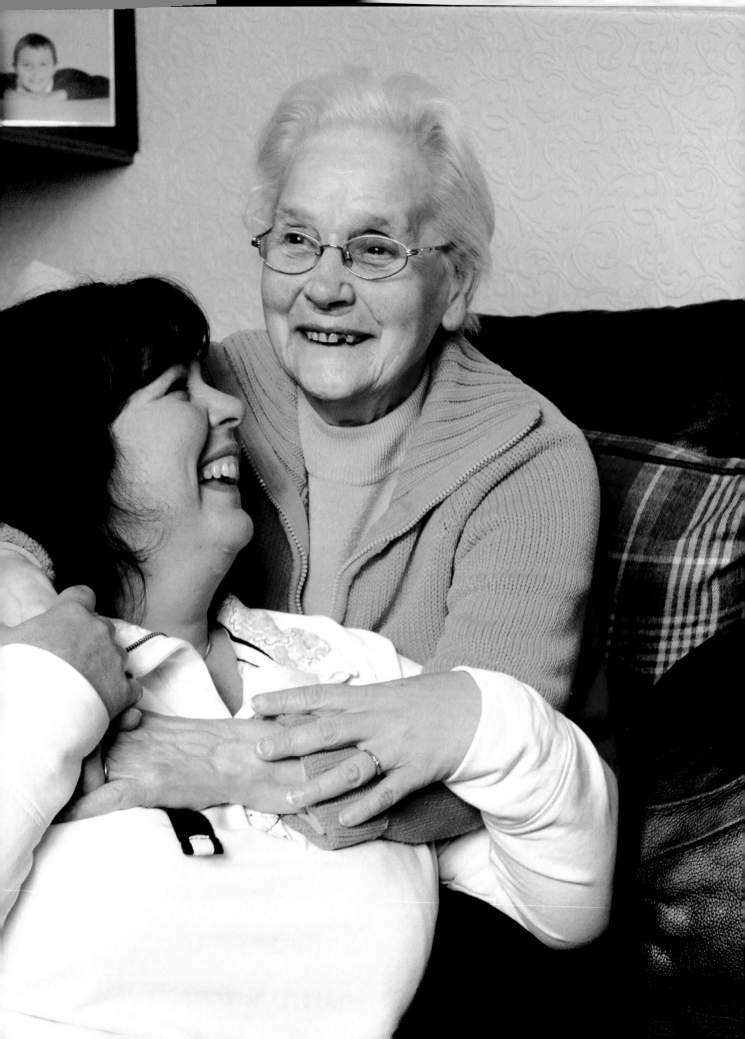

Well-being and response in early stages

Part 3

Chapters

10 Promoting health to reduce risk of dementia

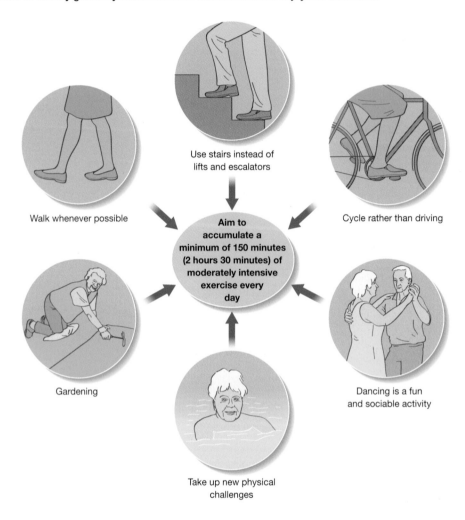

Figure 10.1 Those who have a very sedentary lifestyle should start slowly and build up to higher levels of activity gradually and ensure that the activities are enjoyable and varied

Walk whenever possible

Use stairs instead of lifts and escalators

Cycle rather than driving

Aim to accumulate a minimum of 150 minutes (2 hours 30 minutes) of moderately intensive exercise every day

Gardening

Take up new physical challenges

Dancing is a fun and sociable activity

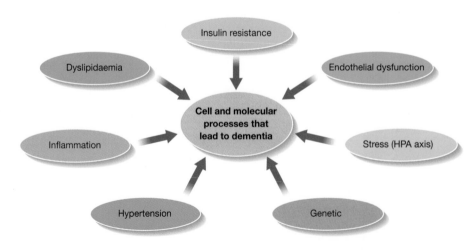

Figure 10. 2 Physiological risk factors that may lead to dementia

Insulin resistance

Dyslipidaemia

Endothelial dysfunction

Cell and molecular processes that lead to dementia

Inflammation

Stress (HPA axis)

Hypertension

Genetic

Dementia Care at a Glance, First Edition. Catharine Jenkins, Laura Ginesi and Bernie Keenan. © 2016 by John Wiley & Sons, Ltd. Published 2016 by John Wiley & Sons, Ltd.
Companion website: www.ataglanceseries.com/nursing/dementiacare

Reducing risk

There is no clear-cut way to prevent dementia but many people are eager to know how to keep their brain sharp as they get older. Dementia is not a normal consequence of ageing, and a compelling body of evidence suggests that lifestyle changes can reduce risk (Figure 10.1). Some forms of dementing diseases take many years to develop, and this is why preventive measures offer hope of reducing their impact.

Everyday physical well-being

Twenty-first century lifestyles and working patterns tend to encourage sedentary behaviour, but the human body was not designed for inactivity. Evidence from large numbers of studies also indicates that paying attention to good nutrition and dental health are key aspect of improving general health and well-being.

Smoking cessation

An important lifestyle factor, the best thing people can do to promote good health and reduce the risk of dementia is to quit smoking. Smoking increases the risk of damage to blood vessels (endothelial dysfunction); it is an important risk factor for stroke and vascular dementia (Chapter 6), both of which affect cognitive processes (Figure 10.2).

Healthier diets

Risk factors that contribute to cardiovascular disease also increase the risk of dementia, so it may be important to cut down intake of meat, high-fat dairy products, fizzy drinks and sweets or candies.

- Limit the amount of salt in the diet to less than 1 teaspoonful (6 grams) per day to reduce the risk of hypertension and stroke.
- Reduce intake of saturated fat – the solid form of fat, which is associated with high levels of cholesterol – to reduce the risk of forming atheromatous plaques, which may contribute to development of vascular dementia.
- Being overweight is associated with higher risk of dementia, and for this reason it is important to maintain calorie balance. This is achieved when calories in the diet are not in excess of calories required by the body for metabolism (cell chemical reactions), growth and physical activity.
- Omega-3 fatty acids (especially docosahexaenoic acid (DHA) and eicosapentaenoic acid (EPA)) are essential for neurocognitive health; these are available from fish and seafood.
- Reduced risk is associated with high intakes of fruit and vegetables, suggesting a key role for antioxidants such as vitamin E, flavonoids and B vitamins.
- The effect of supplementation of vitamins, minerals or ginkgo biloba is unclear, as it may need to be initiated before any detrimental effects begin.
- Tea and coffee drinking may be protective, while too much alcohol is damaging.

Moving more

Physiological benefits of exercise are now well established. They include reduced blood pressure, lowering of levels of 'bad' cholesterol (HDL) in blood and increase in collateral supply of blood to the brain. Such changes may protect from transient ischaemic attacks (TIAs) and stroke. Keeping the body (Figure 10.1) and mind (Chapters 35 and 34) fit and active at any age is therefore an important strategy to reduce the risk of developing dementia – possibly by promoting growth of neurons in the brain. Physical activity is also associated with lower levels of an inflammatory marker known as C-reactive protein; inflammation of the brain has been associated with cognitive decline and greater risk of dementia.

Everyday mental well-being

Cognitive skills are not just about memory and remembering, but include learning, problem-solving and decision-making. It appears to be important to keep challenging the brain to learn new things, thus keeping the mind fit and active right through life. Some positive steps may offer hope of reducing risk and delaying the onset of dementia. There may be an element of mental reserve, which keeps people sharp in their later years. What is not clear is whether intellectual activity promotes a mental reserve that is protective of cognitive decline, or whether some people are biologically at lower risk and have higher mental reserve, thus remaining able to continue cognitive activity for longer.

Thinking and planning

Being mindful – paying attention to the act of doing simple tasks that are familiar like washing up sweeping the floor – is thought to strengthen neural connections. It takes time and effort to live in the moment, but ultimately seems to pay off.

Those who have higher levels of education are at lower risk of dementia so engaging in activities that are intellectually stimulating may be protective. Games like chess, Scrabble, backgammon, bowls and pool – or even driving home by a different route – continually present new challenges. Other activities that promote thinking skills are generally those that engender a feeling of purpose, for example, a rewarding job, playing cards or board games, doing a jigsaw puzzle, gardening and playing musical instruments.

Learning new skills

It is worth bearing in mind that many people find it tricky to take in lots of new information and that everybody's brain ages as they get older. For example, reaction times tend to slow down because brain cells (neurons) do not fire as rapidly as they did in youth. People should be encouraged to try unfamiliar tasks and make the most of opportunities to learn. Human beings are curious creatures and it may be important to introduce an element of adventure or try learning a new language.

Developing social networks

The human brain is designed to interact with other people, and one way of encouraging mental acuity may be to widen your social network. Explaining how things work and engaging in tasks like mentoring young people – whether that may be to teach them how to repair a bicycle or to cook up something special – will keep the brain sharp in older age. Social interactions with others also tend to encourage laughter – another potential protector.

Gendered health

Menopausal women often notice cognitive changes such as forgetfulness that they may report as feeling 'fuzzy' or 'brain fog'. Oestrogen appears to play an important role in modulating sleep and mood and levels of this hormone fall dramatically during menopause.

However, findings about the effectiveness of oestrogen therapy are contradictory and cognitive functions appear to decline at similar rates in men and women.

11 Recognition and assessment

Figure 11.1 More than forgetfulness

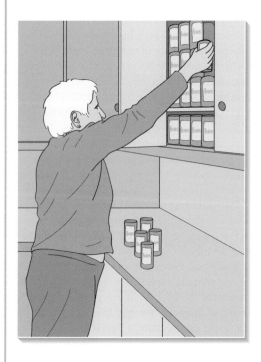

Figure 11.2 MOCA test

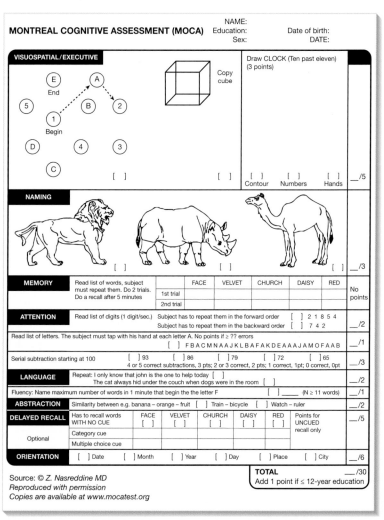

MONTREAL COGNITIVE ASSESSMENT (MOCA)

NAME:
Education:
Sex:
Date of birth:
DATE:

VISUOSPATIAL/EXECUTIVE

Draw CLOCK (Ten past eleven) (3 points)

Copy cube

Contour Numbers Hands ___/5

NAMING

___/3

MEMORY — Read list of words, subject must repeat them. Do 2 trials. Do a recall after 5 minutes

	FACE	VELVET	CHURCH	DAISY	RED	
1st trial						No points
2nd trial						

ATTENTION — Read list of digits (1 digit/sec.) Subject has to repeat them in the forward order [ ] 2 1 8 5 4
Subject has to repeat them in the backward order [ ] 7 4 2 ___/2

Read list of letters. The subject must tap with his hand at each letter A. No points if ≥ ?? errors [ ] F B A C M N A A J K L B A F A K D E A A A J A M O F A A B ___/1

Serial subtraction starting at 100 [ ] 93 [ ] 86 [ ] 79 [ ] 72 [ ] 65
4 or 5 correct subtractions, 3 pts; 2 or 3 correct, 2 pts; 1 correct, 1pt; 0 correct, 0pt ___/3

LANGUAGE — Repeat: I only know that john is the one to help today [ ]
The cat always hid under the couch when dogs were in the room [ ] ___/2

Fluency: Name maximum number of words in 1 minute that begin the the letter F [ ] _____ (N ≥ 11 words) ___/1

ABSTRACTION — Similarity between e.g. banana – orange – fruit [ ] Train – bicycle [ ] Watch – ruler ___/2

DELAYED RECALL — Has to recall words WITH NO CUE

	FACE	VELVET	CHURCH	DAISY	RED	Points for UNCUED recall only	___/5
	[ ]	[ ]	[ ]	[ ]	[ ]		
Optional	Category cue						
	Multiple choice cue						

ORIENTATION [ ] Date [ ] Month [ ] Year [ ] Day [ ] Place [ ] City ___/6

Source: © Z. Nasreddine MD
Reproduced with permission
Copies are available at www.mocatest.org

TOTAL ___/30
Add 1 point if ≤ 12-year education

Figure 11.3 Person being prepared for an MRI scan and MRI scan

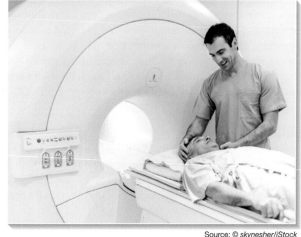

Source: © skynesher/iStock

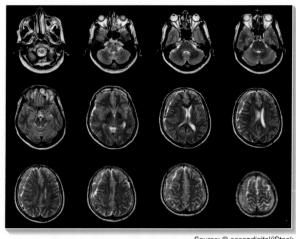

Source: © oceandigital/iStock

Dementia Care at a Glance, First Edition. Catharine Jenkins, Laura Ginesi and Bernie Keenan. © 2016 by John Wiley & Sons, Ltd. Published 2016 by John Wiley & Sons, Ltd.
Companion website: www.ataglanceseries.com/nursing/dementiacare

Forgetfulness

Everyone forgets things sometimes. Most people recognise the feeling of going upstairs to fetch something then, once there, wondering what that something was. When this happens more regularly, people, particularly older people, often fear that this could be a sign of dementia. There is a common assumption that having a poor memory is normal in old age, while a definite diagnosis is often feared. Many people avoid seeing their doctor about memory problems.

Most older people do not have dementia. However, if memory problems are causing difficulties in a person's life, there are good reasons to have an assessment. Many who go to their doctors will be reassured that the problems they experience are normal; for example, it is common to have difficulty concentrating and remembering after bereavement. Some people are found to have a different, treatable problem such as thyroid dysfunction, depression, infection or constipation.

More than forgetfulness – recognising dementia

There are different types of dementia (see Chapters 5–7), so early signs can vary (Figure 11.1). In Alzheimer's type dementia, people will often describe a 'foggy' feeling, that something is wrong, but they cannot explain what. Others will notice they have done slightly odd things, for example putting butter in the microwave instead of the fridge. Friends may tell the person they are repeating themselves. Family may worry the person is not looking after themselves as well as usual. Sometimes people say things that are 'out of character', for example, being 'cheeky' or swearing. People with Lewy body disease may twitch or jerk while sleeping.

When the person with dementia comes back from shopping, they might realise that they have again bought sugar or beans, when they already had plenty in the larder. He or she may find they end up eating the same meal or sandwich every day. Sometimes people get lost in a familiar place, where a small change (e.g. new bus stop) can be very disorientating to them. The person may discover that it is now difficult to follow a TV programme or a novel. If they meet a neighbour on the street, they may realise they cannot remember the person's name. Names of recently bought gadgets (and how they work) may be particularly tricky to recall.

Memory problems are not the only indications of dementia. For some people, their mood becomes very labile, they may feel tearful one minute and cheerful the next. Others find difficulty in judging distance and so have accidents or falls. The problems outlined above usually build up gradually. Within the family, people may make adjustments without realising there is an underlying problem. This can mean that diagnosis is delayed until a crisis happens, for example, if the person gets lost, leaves the gas on or has a car accident. If a person lives alone, they may use various strategies to cope, though others may feel anxious about them.

At present in the United Kingdom, approximately half of people with dementia still do not get a diagnosis. The government has identified changing this as a national priority.

Benefits of diagnosis

The main benefits of diagnosis are access to support, advice and treatment. However, there is also the relief of knowing what the problem is and having the opportunity to plan ahead.

However, for some people, the news is very distressing and can lead to depression and suicidal thinking or actions. For this reason diagnoses should be timely, shared sensitively and never be forced upon a person.

The assessment process

The initial assessment will be carried out by the family doctor who will take a history, take a blood sample to test for treatable causes and carry out a brief memory assessment, such as the '6CIT' or 'mini-mental state examination' (MMSE). The doctor will also have a conversation with the person about their concerns and ask if they would agree to further assessment at a memory clinic.

Memory clinics

Memory clinics are run by mental health professionals working in multi-disciplinary teams who aim to assess whether a person has dementia, what it is caused by or what type it is and then offer treatment, advice and support in coping. A person who is worried about their memory should try to go with a close friend or partner, as they will be able to offer useful additional information to the team and support the person through the process. The psychiatrist or nurse will ask about the history of the problems. They will carry out a memory assessment, using a more detailed assessment tool such as the Montreal Cognitive Assessment (see Figure 11.2). They will do a physical examination and ask about previous health problems and current medications. They will probably offer a scan, such as a CT or MRI (Figure 11.3). After the assessment, the team will share the probable diagnosis with the person and their supporter. They may offer anti-dementia medication and advice on coping strategies, signpost (Chapter 13) to other useful organisations and explain follow-up services. Support will usually involve visits from a community mental health nurse who specialises in the care of people with dementia.

After the diagnosis

Diagnosis provides an indication of the nature of each individual's illness and how it might progress. With this knowledge, it is possible to plan ahead and make decisions about preferences related to care, where to live, how to manage money and so on (Chapter 12). The person can also consider how to live in the moment and make the most of their current abilities and relationships with family and friends. Learning that you have dementia can be an opportunity to meet others in similar situations and develop supportive friendships; it can help to meet people who empathise and share similar experiences to the person and their family. Nowadays, more people open up about living well with dementia and are leading the way in confronting stigma.

12 Post-diagnostic advice

Table 12.1 The advantages and disadvantages of early diagnosis

Advantages of early diagnosis	Disadvantages of early diagnosis
Opportunity to plan ahead	Knowing 'too early' and feeling happy times are overshadowed by fears about the future
Time to talk about the diagnosis openly with friends and family when the person feels ready	Feeling stigmatised, e.g. that other people focus on deficits or no longer take opinions seriously
Time to make legal arrangements for the future	Changing the nature of friendships or losing friends
Access to anti-dementia medication at an early stage, which could slow progression of the condition	Worrying about becoming a 'burden'
Access to local services that provide support for those with dementia	
Access to financial support, e.g. benefits if eligible	
Opportunity to network and gain support from others who are experiencing similar stresses can improve quality of life	
If working in a paid or voluntary role, opportunity to confide in managers and workmates to negotiate adjusted responsibilities	
The chance to take part in changing perceptions and showing that it is possible to 'live well with dementia'	
Opportunity to take steps to maximise health, e.g. exercising, eating healthily	
Understanding that the person 'is not alone' and there is no shame in being diagnosed with the condition	
Being able to continue with normal activities in the knowledge that if they become unsafe others will respond, e.g. with driving	

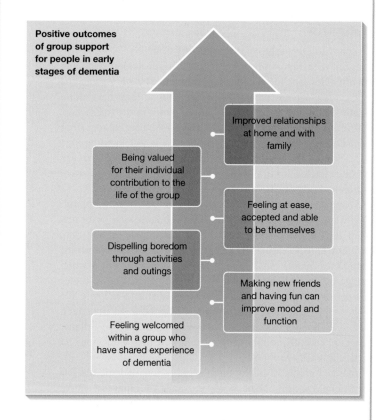

Positive outcomes of group support for people in early stages of dementia

- Improved relationships at home and with family
- Being valued for their individual contribution to the life of the group
- Feeling at ease, accepted and able to be themselves
- Dispelling boredom through activities and outings
- Making new friends and having fun can improve mood and function
- Feeling welcomed within a group who have shared experience of dementia

Table 12.2 Early diagnosis is not right for everyone

- Some people would prefer not to know, whereas others do not feel ready to acknowledge a problem
- Some family doctors do not feel confident in diagnosing dementia

Benefits of delayed diagnosis	Disadvantages of delayed diagnosis
Avoidance of stigma	Missing out on the benefits of early diagnosis outlined in Table 12.1 (left)
No impact on insurance	Family members may become frustrated with the person's perceived repetitiveness or 'laziness' if they do not understand reasons for changes in behaviour
If working, may be able to continue to earn	Family members become stressed by worry or the need to offer support without access to information or support
'Blissful ignorance', avoiding possible shock and depression related to knowing	Being judgemental about oneself and perceived weaknesses
Being able to continue driving, without legal need to inform DVLA	Making dangerous errors when driving a car with potentially catastrophic results

Dementia Care at a Glance, First Edition. Catharine Jenkins, Laura Ginesi and Bernie Keenan. © 2016 by John Wiley & Sons, Ltd. Published 2016 by John Wiley & Sons, Ltd.
Companion website: www.ataglanceseries.com/nursing/dementiacare

Timely diagnosis

People who are diagnosed with dementia have a range of experiences of the assessment and diagnosis process. Some, in line with recent UK government policy, are diagnosed early in the condition and have the news shared sensitively with them. Others may have had symptoms for years before the reason behind them is confirmed. For some it is a relief to have an explanation for the problems, but sometimes the news creates a feeling of bereavement in relation to loss of an expected future and fears about what may lie ahead. The right, or 'timely' moment, for sharing of diagnosis depends on the person. Ideally, they should give informed consent for both the assessment process and hearing the result. Generally, having information at an early stage is perceived as useful by both the person with dementia and their family. It is not good practice to exclude the affected person from discussions of their diagnosis and couples who are able to 'work together' usually fare best as dementia progresses.

Feelings

People who are recently diagnosed may respond with shock, anger, low mood and feelings of hopelessness. However, given support and sensitivity at this time, most people adjust and recognise that it can be empowering to talk about their feelings, plan ahead and adjust to the practicalities of living with dementia. Diagnosis of dementia not only affects the individual with the condition but also has an impact on a whole family network that may need time to express fears and worries, gather information and adjust to the news. Tables 12.1 and 12.2 indicate that the benefits of knowing the diagnosis outweigh the disadvantages for most people, but nevertheless having confirmation of what may have been suspected can be shocking. There is a history of stigmatisation of people with dementia, and most people think of the problems associated with later stages when they consider the term. People in early stages are now more able to 'come out' about the condition and demonstrate what they can continue to do.

Getting support

The person with dementia will need to decide whether and how to tell family and friends about the diagnosis. In many cases, problems will have been noticed by loved ones who may be relieved to know that there is an explanation, even though the diagnosis is concerning. It is never too early to get support and when it is offered people are advised to accept. There is a risk that if help is refused people may not offer again, but once the habit of spending time with the person with dementia is found to be rewarding people are more likely to continue. Even if help is not needed in the initial stages, it can be useful for people with dementia to establish a support network; if or when the condition progresses assistance can be shared and made easier rather than being provided by one or two people only. Health professionals should provide team contact details to make it easy for people with dementia and their relatives to get in touch if advice or support is required.

Understanding the condition

People with dementia can become 'expert patients' in the same way as people with diabetes. Gaining insight into what is happening in the brain can be useful, as it helps people to make sense of memory losses and cognitive changes. Information about common problems and how to manage them is available in leaflet form or online from organisations like the Alzheimer's Society. Voluntary organisations often provide training programmes for people with dementia and family members, and these also offer an opportunity to meet other people who are recently diagnosed.

Practical priorities

Dementia is an age-related condition, and people with dementia often have more than one health problem as they get older. It is a good idea to arrange health checks to ensure that any other health problems are being treated properly, as cognitive symptoms can be worsened by conditions such as poorly controlled diabetes, infection or pain. In addition, it is beneficial to keep dentist and optician's appointments and to explain the diagnosis so that treatment can be arranged while the person is able to give informed consent and professionals can be made aware of the need to provide dementia-friendly explanations and care. A diagnosis of dementia does not need to stand in the way of a full and active life. People with dementia should keep active, eat well and socialise. If they drink alcohol, it is best to do so in moderation. They should continue to enjoy life and contribute to their communities. It is also useful to get in the habit of using a diary, putting keys and other essentials in the same place and having phone numbers written near the phone. Some people choose to carry a card explaining their condition. Reminders can be programmed into mobile devices. Simple assistive technology (see Chapter 44) such as automatic night lights, gas and flood alerts can be purchased in DIY shops.

Planning ahead

It is empowering for people with dementia to make plans for the future and feel reassured that problems are anticipated and solutions prepared to address them in line with their preferences. For example, he or she can explain where and how they would like care to be provided if the need arises. Doing this reduces stress on family members who will not have to guess at a later stage. Younger generations may appreciate learning more about an older person's history and like to help the person with dementia make a life story book which can be used for reminiscence (Chapter 38).

Legal issues

If the person with dementia is a driver, they have a legal responsibility to inform authorities (in the United Kingdom, the DVLA) and their insurance company. They do not necessarily have to give up driving but will need to take a yearly test to ensure that it is safe to carry on.

Under the Mental Capacity Act (2005) (see Chapter 62) people can nominate trusted friends or relatives to have a 'lasting power of attorney' (LPA), which means the nominated person would be responsible for making decisions on the person with dementia's behalf if he/she were no longer able to do so independently. LPAs can be made for financial matters or for health and welfare.

13 Signposting

Figure 13.1 Examples of signposting

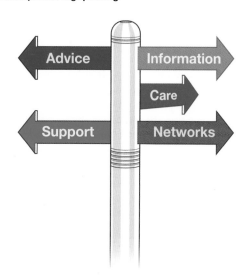

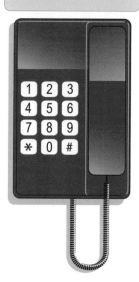

The Alzheimer's Society Helpline:
0300 222 1122

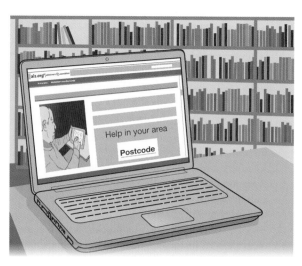

Advice will be available at the doctors surgery, library and at carers support groups

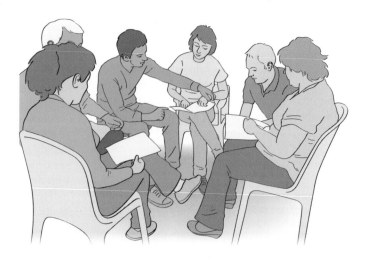

Dementia Care at a Glance, First Edition. Catharine Jenkins, Laura Ginesi and Bernie Keenan. © 2016 by John Wiley & Sons, Ltd. Published 2016 by John Wiley & Sons, Ltd.
Companion website: www.ataglanceseries.com/nursing/dementiacare

The signposting process

Signposting refers to the process of directing people towards further assistance (Figure 13.1). Some sources will be useful across the board, while others may meet the needs of specific groups. Some people may well find themselves on the receiving end of signposting while also looking for further guidance to assist them within their role. This chapter gives information on sources of potential help together with guidance on self-help to aid signposting within local areas. Both Age Action Alliance (http://ageactionalliance.org/) and Dementia Action Alliance (http://www.dementiaaction.org.uk/) have links to a wide range of organisations and telephone contact numbers. Over time, small agencies may have funding withdrawn or merge with others, while new resources could be developed but community hubs such as libraries will hold details of current local resources.

For people diagnosed with dementia

People diagnosed should have access to their own family doctor and practice nurses, plus to a memory clinic. Leaflets about local resources are usually offered, and if they are lost, replacements can be requested. However, after initial diagnosis people are sometimes left wondering what to do next and who to ask for help (Chapter 12).

For a person in this situation, the following will be the main sources of information:

- The Alzheimer's Society: This organisation provides excellent online and printed information, plus sources of support such as befriending services, clubs and telephone advice. They also host online support and chat-rooms.
- Your nearest public library will be able to assist you in finding books about dementia, other information and contact details for the local authority who can provide information about services that they provide directly or fund.
- The GP can make referrals to community walking groups for keeping fit and socialising. Information about these may also be available from the library.
- Social media: If you have Internet access, look for local Facebook pages with links to resources in your area. If there are none suitable, post a message aiming to develop a mutual support network, either online or face to face. Be sure to meet in a public place and tell a trusted friend.
- Age UK. This charity offers advice and support on aspects of living well in old age such as keeping fit, managing finances, including insurance policies and accessing legal advice (e.g. about lasting power of attorney (Chapter 62)) (see http://www.ageuk.org.uk/)
- Your bank. Informing them of your diagnosis will enable them to help you manage your money securely.
- The Driver and Vehicle Licensing Agency (DVLA): It is a legal requirement to inform them of your diagnosis. Depending on medical reports, yearly licenses may be issued (see https://www.gov.uk/government/organisations/driver-and-vehicle-licensing-agency (UK only)).

For people with concerns or 'subjective cognitive impairment'

If you are worried about your memory, you may feel anxious about having an assessment and having those fears confirmed. However, the outcome may be reassuring, or if not, then the diagnosis of dementia, while difficult to come to terms with, is the first step in accessing the support and help you may need now and in future. You may be prescribed anti-dementia medication, which could hold the condition in check and possibly result in some improvement. Sometimes symptoms of dementia are actually related to other, treatable causes, such as thyroid problems or depression, so the best signpost is towards your GP or practice nurse.

If you do not want to see your family doctor (or have done so and been unconvinced by their reassurance), you could request a direct referral to a memory clinic. To do this go online (or to your library and ask for help) and put 'memory clinic' and your area into a search engine. This should result in information on how to get an assessment. Alternatively, look up the local branch of the Alzheimer's society or Citizens' Advice Bureau and arrange an appointment. They will not carry out an assessment but will be able to talk things over with you. It is possible to test your own memory online (http://www.alzheimers.org.uk/). To do this, search for 'Test your Memory' and complete a quiz (http://www.alzheimersreadingroom.com/p/test-your-memory-for-alzheimers-5-best.html). If you are employed, you could approach the Human Resources section, your union and/or occupational health department for advice.

For partners, family and family carers

Professionals should include you in care planning (with your relative's permission) so that you are aware of the services offered and that you are both entitled to. To find out more about dementia, or access further support, you could approach the same organisations listed earlier and:

- The memory clinic who may provide information and training for family carers
- Citizen's Advice Bureaux – for advice on your rights, employment and benefit issues (see http://www.citizensadvice.org.uk/)
- Carers UK who offer information and support for carers (see http://www.carersuk.org/)

For friends of people with dementia

The most important thing is to continue to be present in your friend's life. Understanding more about their experience will help you to make allowances if need be and not take changes in their behaviour personally. You do not need to become a specialist though; including your friend in normal conversations and activities, with small adjustments if necessary, will be best for their well-being. To learn more about dementia, you could become a 'dementia friend' (see http://www.alzheimers.org.uk/ for local sessions) or look at the information provided by the Alzheimer's Society.

For volunteers

You will probably be provided with training, but extra information and guidance can be found on the Alzheimer's Society Website. You could also watch films that give insight into the experiences of people with dementia, such as 'Iris', 'The Iron Lady', 'Still Alice' and 'The Notebook'.

For health professionals

All the previous information should be useful to you. In addition, use the institutional online library and search facilities such as CINAHL and MEDLINE to find specialist recent research-based information. (Librarians will guide you in this process if necessary.) Consider ways of reflecting a person-centred perspective in your work and practice! Further reading could begin with the works of Dawn Brooker, Tom Kitwood and David Sheard.

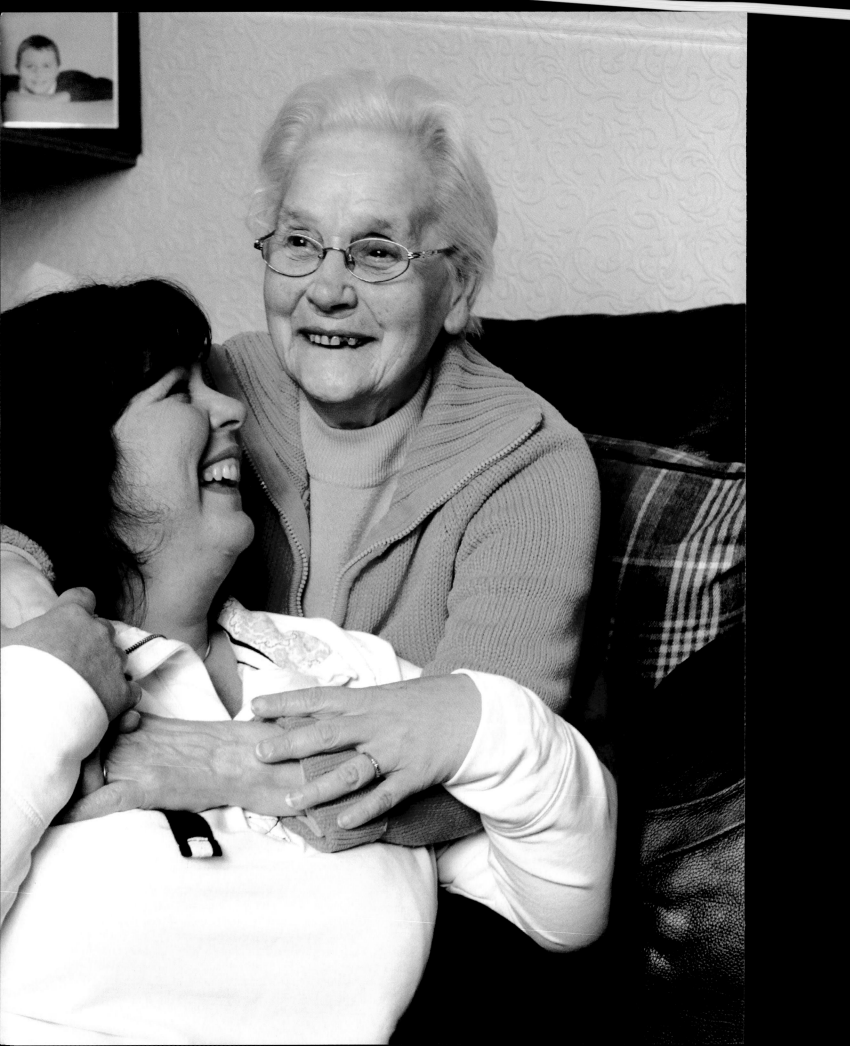

Underpinning principles and skills

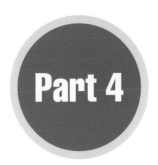

Part 4

Chapters

14 Values: Compassion and dignity

Figure 14.1 Brooker's (2007) work clarifies a strong person-centred approach

V	Valuing the person, regardless of cognitive ability
I	Taking an individual approach
P	Seeing the perspective of each person – putting ourselves in their shoes
S	Considering the social environment – ensuring relationships are supportive

Figure 14.2 The '6 Cs': Values that underpin excellent nursing practice

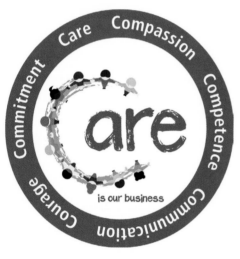

Source: *Reproduced with permission of NHS England*

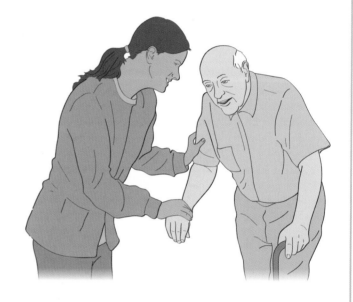

Table 14.1 The '6 Cs' implemented in care

'6 Cs' Value	How they are implemented in the care of people with dementia
Care	Nurses commit to putting the well-being of their patients first and so do whatever they can to promote their health. Care implies concern for a person and action to ensure that their needs are met. Care is not limited to nurses, and people with dementia are also cared for by family members and other health and social care professionals. In the field of dementia care, care may involve listening to someone who is upset, helping them to have a bath or advising family members about local support agencies, among many other activities
Compassion	Compassion is the fellow-feeling that arises when one person meets another who is suffering. It involves feeling sympathetic and motivated to alleviate pain or sorrow. Compassion can be conveyed through facial expression, words and actions
Competence	This is the ability to provide effective interventions. For example, a nurse might prepare for reminiscence sessions by liaising with family members and developing a person-centred reminsinsence box, then demonstrate to colleagues how to use this to engage and interest the service user
Communication	Communication is essential as a basis for interactions with people with dementia, family members and between professionals and others involved in care. Listening is the most important aspect of communiation, but as people with dementia may have impaired communication abilities, nurses and others also need other specific enhanced communication skills (Chapter 18)
Courage	People with dementia sometimes need other people to stand up for their rights and this requires bravery. For example, a nurse may need to argue for higher staffing levels to enable the team to move away from a task orientated approach to a person-centred approach
Commitment	Commitment involves dedication. Caring for people with dementia can be challenging and tiring. Nurses, other professionals, volunteers and family members show commitment in their provision of ongoing support and attention towards people with dementia

Dementia Care at a Glance, First Edition. Catharine Jenkins, Laura Ginesi and Bernie Keenan. © 2016 by John Wiley & Sons, Ltd. Published 2016 by John Wiley & Sons, Ltd.
Companion website: www.ataglanceseries.com/nursing/dementiacare

Values and approaches to care

Values and beliefs are central to the quality of care because of their role in determining a person's approach to caring. Belief that each person is valuable and unique is more likely to guide a family member or professional towards delivering care that is sensitive and person-centred, and a person-centred value system is also likely to increase a carer's job satisfaction. It is important to recognise that each carer has a valuable and unique contribution to make. However, both family and professional carers run the risk of focusing on the well-being of the person with dementia and neglecting their own needs, so respect for values involves respect for and consideration of all parties involved.

All behaviour and communication has meaning

A useful core belief for carers is that everything a person says or does carries a meaning. Sometimes the meaning is not immediately obvious and behaviour may be open to interpretation. It is not always easy to spend time with a person with dementia who may be bored, frightened or frustrated. Sometimes these feelings show in behaviour that can be perceived by others as apathy, attention-seeking or aggression. People who are very dependent on others may feel angry about being so vulnerable. They may appear rude and insensitive or distressed. Carers may need to imagine themselves in the same situation in order to gain insight into these feelings and behaviours. Empathy is also important in imagining how the person's previous experience could be influencing their perception and how, given their disabilities, the world might feel from their perspective. Examining values can help to identify positive approaches to ageing and dementia.

Person-centredness

Person-centred care is a term that sums up care that is designed around an individual, recognising their personality, history, preferences, needs, culture, spirituality and patterns of behaviour and communication (Figure 14.1). It depends on getting to know the person and having a positive approach to solving problems and continuing to develop sensitive care to meet the person's needs. To aid future care, a person and their family can make a life story and complete a form such as the 'All about me' form provided by the Alzheimer's Society so that professionals assisting family members can offer care that is congruent with the norms and wishes of the person. The information included ranges from spiritual beliefs and practices to how the person likes their tea or coffee and how they like to wash and dress. It includes any information and pictures the person would like, for example, photos of family pets.

Empathy

Empathy is a process of imaginatively putting oneself in another's shoes and accurately recognising their emotions. Responding with empathy allows the carer to improve rapport and plan care that meets the emotional as well as the practical needs of the person. Empathy is the basis for comforting compassionate responses and is highly valued by care recipients and family members. Empathic responses show a positive, non-judgemental view of the person. An empathic carer is able to consider the perspective of the person with dementia and the meaning of their behaviour while responding in a warm, supportive manner.

Compassion

When a person responds to suffering with kindness, this indicates compassion. It has been defined as 'intelligent kindness', as the compassionate person uses empathy to identify the struggles and emotions that a person is going through then feels motivated to help them in a way that sensitively anticipates and meets the individual's needs. Compassion has been identified as one of the '6 Cs' of effective caring (Figure 14.2 and Table 14.1).

Dignity

Dignity is at the core of successful, person-centred care. When dignity is promoted and protected, the person with dementia feels safe and well cared-for. Maintaining privacy, giving personal care in a sensitive way, protecting the person from discrimination and negative interactions or abuse, maintaining self-esteem, communicating sensitively and respectfully (not contradicting), enabling choice and autonomy and recognizing and including the individual all contribute to provision of care that supports dignity.

Respect

Respect results from positive feelings towards another person. Rudeness and lack of consideration indicate lack of respect and lead to feelings of humiliation and poor self-esteem. People with dementia rely more on others' responses to them in order to maintain their identity and self-esteem, so respectful interactions are a cornerstone of person-centred care and protecting personhood.

Positive attitudes and mutual respect within the care team are similarly essential in promoting cooperation, continuity and consistency. Sometimes people with dementia do not convey respect for others. It is difficult for them to empathise with others, as they do not always understand the constraints within which people are working or correctly identify relationships. If a person with dementia behaves rudely, it is important for care teams to remember this and respond calmly, explaining the situation clearly sensitively and non-judgmentally.

Protection

Autonomy and choice may need to be balanced with protection as a person's dementia progresses. Professional and family carers will gradually take on responsibility for keeping the person safe. Abuse of any sort should never be tolerated and appropriate safeguarding measures taken if necessary (Chapter 59).

Comfort, well-being and enjoyment of life

People with dementia need to feel secure within a group. Having fun, laughing, taking part in meaningful activities and enjoying relationships all contribute to well-being. People with dementia are able to give care as well as to receive it, and mutuality in warm, positive relationships should be acknowledged and welcomed.

15 The work of Tom Kitwood

Figure 15.1 Social psychology

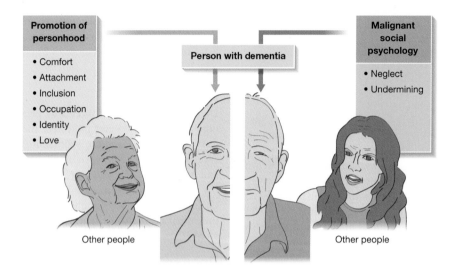

Table 15.1 Examples of malignant social psychology

Treachery	Betraying the trust of the person with dementia, for example tricking them into doing something by lying
Disempowerment	Doing things for the person when it is not necessary, leading to them losing skills and independence
Infantilisation	Treating a person with dementia as if they were a child, talking to them in baby language
Intimidation	Deliberately frightening the person so that they comply with others' wishes
Labelling	Referring to people only in terms of their diagnosis, rather than as individuals
Outpacing	Doing things at the pace of the carer, rather than making reasonable adjustments so that the person with dementia can keep up and retain control and involvement
Invalidation	Perceiving everything the person with dementia says or does as a symptom of dementia, rather than seeing them as an individual with legitimate opinions
Objectification	Treating people as objects around which tasks have to be performed, such as feeding and washing. Not taking the person's experience into account
Disruption	Interrupting what a person is doing because it is not seen as valuable or significant
Mockery and disparagement	Teasing a person, or saying negative undermining things which damage their sense of self

Table 15.2 Positive interactions that promote personhood

Recognition	Interacting with a person acknowledging who they are, their preferences, life history, use of language
Collaboration	Doing activities together, supporting them in joining in and being active participants
Play	Having fun, doing things they enjoy
Celebration	Marking an occasion identifying achievements, recognising positive events publically
Relaxation	Acknowledging and using time to sit back and unwind
Validation	Recognising emotions and reflecting back to the person that they are real, heard and acknowledged
Holding	Providing a safe space and relationships where the person feels secure
Facilitation	Enabling the person to be included through use of sensitive communication and environmental adjustments

Dementia Care at a Glance, First Edition. Catharine Jenkins, Laura Ginesi and Bernie Keenan. © 2016 by John Wiley & Sons, Ltd. Published 2016 by John Wiley & Sons, Ltd.
Companion website: www.ataglanceseries.com/nursing/dementiacare

Tom Kitwood: Dementia Care Pioneer

Tom Kitwood (1937–1998) was hugely influential in promoting a person-centred approach to the care of people with dementia. Writing and practising in the 1980s and 1990s, he challenged the therapeutic nihilism of the time which he called the 'old culture of dementia care'. This had resulted in 'one-size-fits-all' care in which the needs of individuals with dementia were not recognised and in which those with dementia were not valued, listened to or included. People were often cared for with little concern for privacy, for example, all lining up to go to the toilet after meals, their days timetabled around the needs of the organisation providing care, with little engagement or activity. Unfortunately, there are still some instances of these practices, and Kitwood's messages, while forceful, are not always heard by health and social care professionals. Research and training approaches are continuing to explore how his philosophy can be developed, applied and expanded so that sensitive, person-centred care can be offered to all with dementia who may need it.

Kitwood's life

Tom Kitwood was born in Lincolnshire, UK, in 1937. He graduated from Cambridge before training for the priesthood. After National Service, he taught chemistry in Dorset and later in Uganda, where he was also a school chaplain. On return to the United Kingdom, he settled in Bradford, where he completed MSc and PhD degrees at Bradford University. In 1984 he became a senior lecturer in psychology there, specialising in psychogerontology and dementia care, founding the Bradford Dementia Group and subsequently being appointed Professor. He retained a spiritual outlook, though with a humanistic rather than Christian focus later in his life. He wrote many papers on the person-centred approach. His most famous work, 'Dementia reconsidered: the person comes first' was published in 1997. He developed a means of evaluating care from the perspective of the experience of the person with dementia in the form of Dementia Care Mapping (DCM). He also developed training courses in person-centred care approaches. Tom Kitwood was a warm, charismatic and engaging person whose ideas have influenced the field of dementia care all over the world. Sadly, he died in 1998.

Kitwood's ideas

Defining dementia

Within the old culture of dementia care, dementia was seen as a result of neurological damage. Kitwood challenged this medicalised view by taking the perspective of the person's experience. While acknowledging that neuropathic change plays a part, he broadened the definition of dementia to include aspects such as the person's history, personality and the social environment in which they live.

He made this definition into an equation, so that Dementia = Personality + Biography + Health + Neurological Impairment + Social Psychology, with all factors seen to interact with each other.

Malignant social psychology

Kitwood believed that neurological impairment in an older person attracted what he termed 'malignant social psychology' (MSP). Social psychology refers to the nature of the relationships with others. He noted that people with dementia were often ignored, excluded and objectified and their attempts to communicate and be involved with others overlooked or rejected. He went on to suggest that this process led to further neurological damage and impairment. Thus, MSP contributes to the process of deterioration in the person's functioning and well-being in a negative spiral. He listed the damaging interactions that should be avoided (see Table 15.1).

Personhood

Kitwood defined his central concept of Personhood as 'a standing or status bestowed on one human being, by others, in the context of relationship and social being. It implies recognition, respect and trust' (1997:8). In the same way that malignant interactions can damage a person, positive interactions can support, protect and, even in some cases, improve the person's condition, a process he called 'rementia'. This concept is hugely meaningful for those giving care to people with dementia, as it highlights the impact of positive interactions and the responsibilities of care workers to take care to relate to people with dementia in ways that enhance a sense of self. Kitwood suggested that the psychological needs of people with dementia are for inclusion, acceptance, attachment, comfort, identity and love. He recommended positive interactions that can contribute to meeting these needs (see Table 15.2).

Dementia care mapping

DCM is the method Kitwood developed for evaluating the care of people with dementia in formal settings such as care homes. Trained observers note well-being (personal enhancers) and ill-being (personal detractors) through frequent recording of interactions and activities and interpreting behavioural signs. Mapping only takes place in public areas. Results reflect the extent to which emotional needs (as in Figure 15.1) have been met, and these can be used to provide feedback to staff on good practice, gaps in care and training needs.

Critiquing Kitwood

Kitwood died while still developing his theories and no doubt would have continued to refine his ideas. His writings are rather philosophical and have been criticised for being difficult to understand for many who work in hands-on care. His evidence base has also been challenged as his theories are mainly based on unpublished work and anecdotal reports. Kitwood's definitions do not really allow two-way relationships for people with dementia; they are seen as recipients rather than people with degrees of autonomy. In addition, the concept of MSP may unfairly implicate carers in a person's decline when they are doing their best in difficult circumstances. However, despite these issues, Kitwood's work continues to inspire others and drive positive, person-centred approaches to care.

16 Cultural issues

Table 16.1   Cultural definitions

Ethnicity	Belonging to a group of people with a shared geographical, ancestral, linguistic and cultural tradition
Race	Belonging to a population with shared genetically determined physical characteristics, e.g. skin tone. The scientific evidence for 'race' is weak
Culture	Shared beliefs and way of life in a society

Figure 16.1   Iceberg diagram

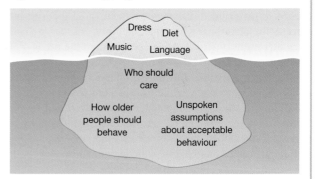

Table 16.2   Cultural dimensions and their implications

Hofstede's cultural dimensions	Explanation: The extent to which ...	Implications for dementia care
Power – distance	People accept hierarchy or value equality	Stronger power distance families (who accept hierarchy) find it easier to take advice from a professional if they are aware of their qualifications and experience. Weaker power distance families prefer a more collaborative, jointly developed care plan
Individualism/collectivism	Someone sees themselves primarily as part of their tight-knit group or as an independently functioning individual	Decisions about care may be seen as family matters or the person and immediate carer may be responsible for independent decision-making
Uncertainty avoidance	People feel comfortable or uncomfortable with ambiguity and the unknown	People may ask for all possible information relating to dementia so as to plan ahead, or they may prefer to wait and see whether problems develop
Masculinity/feminity	People value competitiveness and achievements or cooperation and mutual concern	It may be difficult to cope with the changing abilities of the person with dementia, or the person may be included by family and friends, with less judgement made about their disabilities

Box 16.1   Pointers for positive transcultural care practices

- Be aware of your own feelings and responses; reflect upon the meaning of these and the impact they could have on a person from a different cultural background
- Avoid assumptions (e.g. that some families will want to care for a person at home, while others will want a care home)
- Get to know families and individuals – if not sure about cultural norms, ask
- Show warmth and friendliness
- Be aware of essential religious and cultural aspects of care (e.g. diet, clothing, gender of carer) and adjust care accordingly

Table 16.3   Transcultural communication

Language	• Learn some greetings and words in your clients' languages • Avoid relying on family members to translate except in emergencies • Consultations involving interpreters take at least twice as long as without
Individual differences	• Respect others' expectations about privacy and confidentiality if requested • People may need more, or less, personal space than you are used to • Eye contact norms may be different from your own
Make sure that you	• Avoid making assumptions about motives • Convey respect, e.g. through language and gestures • Are prepared to be flexible with time, e.g. your client may work to a diary or be more flexible in their understanding

Box 16.2   Top tips for working with an interpreter

- Make sure they speak the right language!
- Interpreters should be paid professionals (not family members and especially not children)
- Allow plenty of time – everything will have to be said at least twice
- Be sensitive to diversity issues – for example ask for an interpreter of the same gender as the client and from the same ethnic group
- Prepare the interpreter in advance about the purpose of the meeting
- Ask them to tell you exactly what the person says
- Ask them to confirm with the client that the conversation is confidential
- Ensure you sit equally spaced and direct your conversation towards the client
- Express yourself clearly, stop between sentences and avoid jargon
- Support the interpreter if the content of the conversation is upsetting
- Re-book the same interpreter if their rapport with the client was good

Dementia Care at a Glance, First Edition. Catharine Jenkins, Laura Ginesi and Bernie Keenan. © 2016 by John Wiley & Sons, Ltd. Published 2016 by John Wiley & Sons, Ltd.
Companion website: www.ataglanceseries.com/nursing/dementiacare

The significance of culture

The term 'culture' refers to the norms and values that we take for granted but which nevertheless guide how we live our lives (Table 16.1). As individuals, our norms seem ordinary and obvious because they are familiar, which is why other people's cultures may seem more visible than our own. However, all groups have cultures. Groups of people may come together through shared geographical location, ethnicity, education, membership of a minority group (e.g. through sexual orientation, disability, religious belief), professional values, political ideology, shared hobby and so on. Most of us are members of more than one group, so we become used to adjusting our language and behaviour accordingly. Understanding cultural issues is particularly relevant to dementia care because cultural values guide beliefs, attitudes and behaviours around old age, what we believe dementia is and how we feel care should be given and received (Table 16.2 and Box 16.1).

Healthcare professionals are usually able to articulate the belief systems that guide their interventions, but that is less often the case for individuals and families, mainly because shared attitudes are generally acted on and reinforced rather than discussed. Members of a majority culture find their own attitudes reflected in everyday life and in the media, which makes them feel 'normal', while minority groups are likely to become more aware of differences. There are more differences within groups than between them and membership of a group does not determine the attitude or belief of an individual. It is good to accept that we are all different in some respects while being similar in others. Acculturation is the process of adjusting to another culture, and as individuals and members of groups, we can learn from each other and choose to change if we wish.

Culture and old age

Cultural values and beliefs underpin many attitudes that are relevant to understanding old age and how people with dementia should be cared for (Figure 16.1), for example:

• When old age begins, that is any age between 50 and 80 years.
• Ideas about suitable behaviour for older men and women, for example, suitable dress, whether the older person should now sit back and put their feet up, take a leading role in making family decisions, retire or carry on working or provide child care.
• The causations of mental illness, for example, genetics, bad luck, social deprivation, spiritual disharmony or 'karma' and unhealthy lifestyle.
• The role of the sick person – should they fight their illness or allow themselves to be cared for?
• Who should be a carer, for example, family member or professional?
• Whether to wash in a bath or running water as in a shower.

Not all cultural expectations are fulfilled; for example, many older people find themselves taking on the challenging role of becoming carer for their partner at a time when they would have expected to take life more easily. Cultural values also determine, to some extent, a person's status within their family. The judgement of older people may be deferred to, or alternatively, particularly within ageist societies, older peoples' views may be dismissed. It is difficult for someone brought up to value elders to find they are not so valued in turn by acculturated younger generations. Ageist values in Western societies can combine with stigma towards dementia so that people with dementia are excluded and devalued. Those from minority groups may experience multiple jeopardy; for example, when ageism, anti-dementia stigma and racism and/or homophobia combine so that they are further disadvantaged.

Memory problems and cultural responses

Defining the range of experiences associated with poor memory in someone getting old as a condition, syndrome or disease in itself reflects cultural values. Dementia is generally perceived as a syndrome (collection of symptoms caused by a disease process) by health and social care professionals. However, many lay people from a variety of cultural backgrounds believe memory problems are to be expected in old age. Unfortunately, people have been occasionally denied assessment and access to treatment by healthcare professionals who are more influenced by lay beliefs than professional training. Viewing the experience of dementia as natural may be positive for inclusion within the family network, but there is a risk that the affected person's needs are ignored or behaviour interpreted as a form of 'madness'. Lack of recognition of dementia as a specific condition can exacerbate stigma, lead to denial, further exclusion from society and undermine access to services.

The difficulties associated with progression of memory problems are themselves open to culturally driven perceptions. Disinhibited language and behaviour may be judged as inappropriate and the person's standing within the family undermined. Repetitive questioning, non-recognition of family members and difficulties with personal hygiene are all likely to transgress cultural norms and may cause distress to others. As language skills reduce, the person with dementia may use formerly acceptable terms (e.g. 'spastic') considered unacceptable nowadays. He/she may behave according to their previous cultural norms and behave in ways now seen as sexist or racist. He/she may believe they live in a former time and place, which can be confusing and undermining for loved ones, for example a gay partner in an 'out', committed relationship may misinterpret their partner's apparent denial (an essential survival tactic in former times). A youth-orientated value system and less contact with birth families can isolate older gay couples.

Culture and care

Cultural values also guide individual's beliefs about who should care for people with dementia. In most traditional societies, there is an assumption that caring is 'women's work'. This may be a wife, daughter, daughter-in-law or paid carer. In more collective societies, caring is shared (though the role may still fall mainly on one person), whereas in individualist societies professional care is usually more acceptable, although most people are still cared for at home by a (female) family member. Caring may be seen as a burden or as a rewarding duty and opportunity to repay a caring debt. Healthcare professionals need to develop awareness about their own cultural beliefs. It is important to remain non-judgemental and supportive when a family approaches the person with dementia in a way that is different from one's own. If unsure, the best approach is to keep an open mind, ask, listen, learn and adjust, maintaining a positive rapport with the person with dementia and their family members (Tables 16.3 and Box 16.2).

17 Spirituality

Figure 17.1 Spirituality has different meanings for different people

For many people, feeling connected to the natural world is central to their spiritual well-being

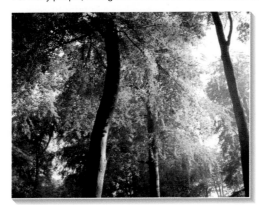
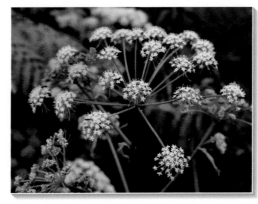

For others, it is important to be part of a faith community and to meet others in a religious context

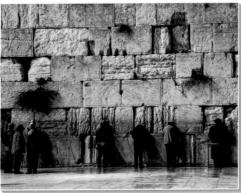
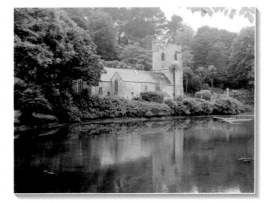

Source: © AndreyKrav/iStock

Table 17.1 Spiritual care plan example

Care planning for spiritual needs ensures they are not forgotten and clarifies expectations for care staff.
They should be written together with the person with dementia and/or people who know them well.

Spiritual need	Aim	Action	Responsible person
Betty is a Christian. She needs to worship by praying independently and together with her congregation. She has forgotten some of the prayers but remembers traditional hymns	Betty will be able to worship at home and continue to attend church and remain connected to friends there, so as to meet her spiritual needs	• Staff members to support Betty in using her prayer book every evening • Liaise with the minister about suitable services and volunteer transport • Discuss with Betty whether she would like religious pictures or items in her room to orientate and comfort her • Use TV programmes (and recordings) that feature worship to enable Betty to feel connected on days she does not go to church	Nurses, carers, church members, family members
Jonas has always loved being outdoors and mountain climbing. He likes to feel connected to nature	Jonas will have opportunities to be outside and to walk in fresh air	• Staff members to arrange a walk in green spaces twice weekly • Support Jonas in expressing feelings about this • Put Jonas' mountaineering photos on a DVD and play weekly on his TV • Talk with him about his travels and adventures	Friends and family, nurses and carers

Dementia Care at a Glance, First Edition. Catharine Jenkins, Laura Ginesi and Bernie Keenan. © 2016 by John Wiley & Sons, Ltd. Published 2016 by John Wiley & Sons, Ltd.
Companion website: www.ataglanceseries.com/nursing/dementiacare

Defining spirituality

Spirituality has different meanings for different people, but 'meaning' is central to the idea of how spirituality is relevant to life (Figure 17.1). For some people, spirituality is aligned with a particular religion or belief system, while for others the 'meaning' comes from a relationship with nature, a sense of being part of a pattern within the universe, feeling moved by art or music or dedicating their life to a cause or to the well-being of others. People with dementia, in common with other people, have a wide variety of spiritual expressions and experiences. Even within a traditional faith community each individual's experiences and beliefs vary. Whatever the nature of a person's spirituality, it involves:

• A sense of connectedness – this could be to a deity or deities, to the natural world and/or to other people
• A sense of purpose – the person's beliefs guide and influence their behaviour
• A sense of transcendence or awe – a feeling of wonder, of being at peace and emotionally in tune with the moment

These aspects combine to create spiritual meaningfulness in a person's life.

A sense of the spiritual may occur individually or in a group. For many it involves worship and being part of a faith community who support each other and within which guidance is offered. The community may have expectations of the behaviour of its members and encourage them to comply, for example, with dress, diet, relationship and other norms for the common good. Faith communities aim to act with compassion towards their members and others, guided by belief that their deity or prophets indicate that this is positive for their own and others well-being and afterlife.

Spirituality and living with dementia

Living in the moment

The nature of dementia means that people may have strengths that make them more connected to others and develop more appreciation of the small details of life. Small moments, for example, in the company of a small child, or reminiscing about happy times, or being in a garden, clearly bring great joy.

Potential crises related to spiritual needs

Unfortunately, the times of joy are often out-weighed by difficulties that cause great distress. The connections to others that are so essential for the person with dementia's well-being can be overwhelming and exhausting for others. Even with excellent care, there is a risk that in later stages a person will feel lonely or abandoned; having no memory of the recent visit of a loved one.

Spiritual needs vary not only according to the individual and their personal beliefs but also in relation to their current stage and experience of dementia. In the early stages, people may fear what lies ahead, of losing aspects of their personhood or of not being able to offer meaning through their own contributions. They may fear losing a relationship with God or a higher being, or not being able to take part in rituals of worship. Sometimes dementia is interpreted as a punishment from God or related to 'karma' and past misdeeds and so may be accompanied by guilt

or shame. In later stages a person may feel unable to worship independently, may miss the comfort of prayer and ceremony, and feel unable to articulate what is meaningful to them. Alternative expressions of spirituality, for example, closeness to mature or helping others, may become more difficult to address as dementia progresses, due to difficulties with access.

Health and social care professionals

Professionals often worry about including spiritual needs in assessments and care plans because of concerns about offending people, being seen as attempting to influence service users or feeling inadequate or inexperienced in coping with spiritual issues. These anxieties are best approached honestly and directly, by asking the person, as part of a normal conversation, about their beliefs, values and spiritual and religious practices, with the aim of providing sensitive, person-centred care. Spiritual care also includes the spiritual needs of those who are not religious. Personal approaches to spirituality should be included within life stories. If spiritual needs are acknowledged in care plans, it is more likely that they will be met (Table 17.2).

The 'golden rule'

Certain principles are similarly expressed in the traditions of the world's great religions, for example, to consider the needs of our neighbours as equal to our own and to do to others what we would wish for ourselves. This principle is relevant to people with dementia who are our spiritual neighbours (and actual neighbours too). Most people would probably prefer to continue to feel welcomed and accepted by their communities and to have opportunities to take part in activities that make life worthwhile and give it meaning.

Responses of faith communities

Spontaneous worship can become more difficult for people with dementia, as can long ceremonies or rituals. However, people value being included in congregations and having the opportunity to belong to their group and to worship with others. Adjustments to ceremonies, while keeping the essence can enable those with disabilities, including dementia, to remain observant. Adjustments could include:

• Linking spiritual values to the needs of people with dementia
• Simplified services, slower paced
• Inclusion of familiar music and traditional wordings
• Modelling acceptance, welcome and care
• Orientating the person to the ritual, for example, by praying alongside them and providing written versions of prayers
• Reinforcing central messages of faith and love
• Encouragement of active support by congregation members, for example, in providing transport, accompanying to worship and directing to toilet facilities
• Welcoming the contributions of people with dementia
• Committing to being a dementia-friendly faith community

Spiritual needs should be considered within all environments so that people with dementia can experience a sense of awe, find meaning in life, give to others and accept help themselves, while feeling connected, loved, significant and valued.

18 Communication

Box 18.1 Communication difficulties

Early stages

- Word-finding problems
- Repetitiveness
- Difficulty remembering and understanding 'new' words, or jargon
- Less spontaneity in speech

Middle stages

- Difficulty in expressing ideas
- Circumlocution (convolutedness)
- Reduced use of nouns
- Difficulty understanding complex sentences
- Poor concentration
- Repetitiveness
- May use the 'wrong' word or a word that has similar meaning or sound

Later stages

- Conversation may be very difficult to follow
- Reduced use of vocabulary
- Difficulty with names and nouns
- May repeat the same phrases
- Sentences very disjointed; speech difficult or impossible to follow
- May get very frustrated by communication difficulties
- May echo what is said
- Eventually not able to speak but may make incomprehensible sounds

Figure 18.1 Areas of the brain responsible for language processing include Wernicke's area, Broca's area and motor cortex

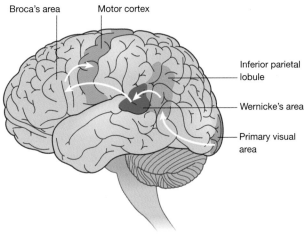

Broca's area   Motor cortex

Inferior parietal lobule

Wernicke's area

Primary visual area

Wernicke's area interprets words we hear or read and then relays information to Broca's area, which generates words or speech in response

The inferior parietal lobule (Geschwind's territory) lies at a key junction between the visual, auditory and somato-sensory cortex, so its neurons respond to many different kinds of inputs. This part of the brain is thought to be involved in many different types of neural operations including sensory integration, spatial attention and oculomotor control and may therefore help us to label and classify things – a skill that is needed for abstract thinking

Box 18.2 Top tips

- Use short sentences, familiar words, repetition and a calm friendly tone
- Allow time for the person with dementia to take in what you say
- Use 'cues', e.g. by including context such as peoples' names, the time, location and subtle reminding of conversational subject
- Avoid unnecessary questions and contradicting the person
- Avoid 'elderspeak' – talking to the person as if they were a child (being patronising and using an unnaturally high pitch)
- Do make decisions easy, e.g. 'Let's watch TV. Do you like sports?'

Figure 18.2 Things to remember

- Take time to make contact
- Listen
- Adjust your speech to the person's abilities
- Enjoy the company of the person

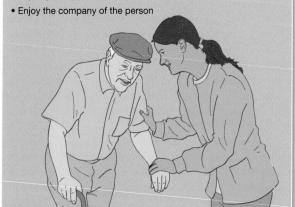

Dementia Care at a Glance, First Edition. Catharine Jenkins, Laura Ginesi and Bernie Keenan. © 2016 by John Wiley & Sons, Ltd. Published 2016 by John Wiley & Sons, Ltd.
Companion website: www.ataglanceseries.com/nursing/dementiacare

In the early stages of dementia, most people will be able to communicate effectively using their usual mediums of spoken and written language and gesture, and will be able to understand other people (Figure 18.1). Occasional word-finding difficulties are common but do not prevent the person from managing their life and relating to other people. More sophisticated language, such as that used in legal or technical documents, can become difficult to follow, while recently learnt vocabulary or means of communication, such as social media (e.g. Facebook, Snapchat, Audioboom) may become difficult to keep up with, as they are for a lot of people who do not have dementia.

As the condition progresses, the person with dementia may gradually find it difficult to make sense of long sentences or complex grammatical structures (Figure 18.1). For example, double negatives ('that's not a bad idea') or subordinate clauses (if… then…) can be confusing. Later in the condition, word finding of everyday vocabulary also becomes difficult leading to problems expressing thoughts and feelings, which can be frustrating for people with dementia and upsetting for their family and friends. The person with dementia will also find understanding other people increasingly difficult. Communication difficulties are related to the causation of dementia, but skilled communication techniques can significantly mitigate the effects and enable people with dementia to feel understood and connected to others as the dementia progresses.

The brain and communication

Communication difficulties are caused by damage to the language-related pathway(s) of the cerebral cortex that deal with perception, memory, comprehension and production of language (see Figure 18.1). Inputs relating to words and sounds (auditory cortex) or written codes, sign language and images (visual cortex) are normally processed in the temporal lobe (including **Wernicke's area**). This part of the brain is responsible for understanding of language; degeneration of Wernicke's area results in vocabulary difficulties – usually in finding the right word. The **arcuate fasciculus** connects with **Broca's area** (frontal lobe) whose function is the production of meaningful language.

In turn, speech information is normally relayed on (transcoded) to the **motor cortex** and other areas responsible for muscle movements necessary for speaking or writing. Thus, lesions in Broca's area lead to difficulties with syntax (grammar, the patterns of how words work together). In most types of dementia, there is a gradual deterioration in the person's ability to express themselves and to understand other people.

Communication approach

Successful communication is based on interest, empathy, patience and a caring approach (Figure 18.2). People with dementia need others to make adjustments to their communication styles to compensate for dementia-related disability and to offer reassurance and kindness to help them cope with their emotions. It is important to try to understand the person as much as possible so that the approach to communication is appropriate for building on strengths while minimising impact of weaknesses. Knowing the person also helps with topics of conversation, knowing their worries and what reassures them. Spending time with a person communicates to them that they are important. It is most beneficial to include the person in conversations and let them know that they are valued, welcome and recognised for who they are.

Listening

Orientation, concentration, short-term memory problems and word-finding difficulties mean people with dementia often struggle to convey thoughts, wishes and feelings. Listening can be difficult and sometimes people without dementia are tempted to avoid those with dementia. However, this is not a solution because of the negative emotional impact on the person and because not listening can lead to frustration, sadness and neglect. Effective listening is essential in meeting the practical and emotional needs of people with dementia and it involves:

- Observing facial expression and body language
- Hearing and making effort to understand the content of speech
- Showing you are interested by drawing near, being at the same level, smiling, leaning forward and taking turns in conversation
- Checking understanding by repeating the gist of what the person has said in question form
- Suggesting words if they have been forgotten
- Responding to feelings, even when facts are unclear
- Noticing behaviour that may communicate unmet need, such as pain or to go to the toilet

Non-verbal communication

Clear body language can assist the person with dementia in understanding others. Facial expressions convey feelings, gestures can reinforce meanings. It is important to be congruent with non-verbal and verbal communication so as to avoid mixed messages. Gentle touch can be helpful if it feels appropriate. The context of communication helps, for example, being near a tea pot and pointing at it, while lifting an imaginary cup, eyebrows raised in question, would help convey the message of offering tea.

Verbal communication

Use of words needs to be clear and specific. It is important to call the person with dementia by their preferred name and remind them of other people's names if necessary. Nouns, which are the subject of a sentence, are best near the beginning of a sentence because they focus attention appropriately and clarify intention. For example, it is better to say 'put your bottom on the chair' rather than 'please sit down'. Warmth and friendliness should be conveyed through smiling and tone of voice.

Communicating without language

When a person's language is severely damaged, they benefit more than ever from human interaction. Use of gentle reassuring touch, smiles, eye contact and warm words will help them feel safe. Even if it is not possible to understand what the person with dementia is saying, or he/she is not able to say anything, it is important to aim to understand the feeling they express and respond accordingly.

19 Common dementia-related problems

Table 19.1 An example of part of an 'ABC' chart

Antecedent (what happens beforehand)	Behaviour (description of incident or problem)	Consequence (what happens afterwards)
The doctor called to visit Geoff, so Nick went to get him out of bed earlier than his usual time and in a bit of a rush	Geoff refused to get out of bed, and when Nick approached, he tried to kick him	The doctor offered to prescribe some medication to address Geoff's behaviour, but Nick suggested that rushing Geoff had upset him and it was not necessary

Table 19.2 Possible causes of agitation

Environment
- Lack of stimulation
- Over-stimulation
- Sensory deprivation
- Lack of exercise
- Too noisy
- Too dark
- Exhaustion

Psychological
- Feeling overwhelmed
- Needs not being met
- Reduced ability to communicate
- Malignant social psycholgical (see Chapter 15)

Aggravated responses
- Psychotrophic medication
- Inappropriate restraint

Figure 19.1 Four categories of agitated behaviour

1 Aggressive behaviour
- Hitting
- Biting
- Kicking
- Pushing
- Scratching
- Tearing things
- Cursing

2 Physically non-aggressive behaviour
- Pacing and restlessness
- Handling things inappropriately
- Trying to get to a different place
- Repititious mannerisms
- Inappropriate robing/disrobing
- Rocking

3 Verbally agitated behaviour
- Continual requests for attention,
- Complaining
- Negativity
- Repititious questions
- Being afraid

4 Hiding and hoarding behaviour
- Attempting to keep valuables safe
- Rummaging for things
- Emotional attachment to objects that may appear worthless

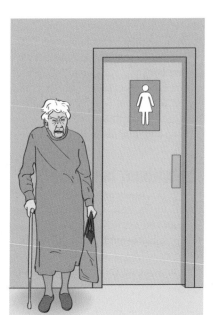
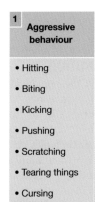

Figure 19.2 The needs of people with dementia according to Kitwood (1997) – see Chapter 15

It can be useful to consider whether the behaviour of a person with dementia reflects an 'unmet need' and if steps could be taken to meet this need. Unmet needs include those for physical health care, e.g. pain relief or treatment of an infection

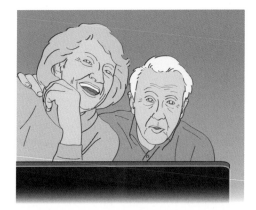
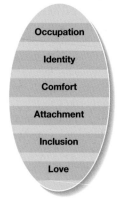

Occupation
Identity
Comfort
Attachment
Inclusion
Love

Dementia Care at a Glance, First Edition. Catharine Jenkins, Laura Ginesi and Bernie Keenan. © 2016 by John Wiley & Sons, Ltd. Published 2016 by John Wiley & Sons, Ltd.
Companion website: www.ataglanceseries.com/nursing/dementiacare

Why difficulties arise

Memory problems and other difficulties associated with dementia can lead to a variety of issues:

- Language problems may cause difficulties in self-expression and understanding others leading to frustration or withdrawal.
- Disorientation can lead to anxiety and the need for reassurance.
- Not being able to follow a sequence of actions to achieve an objective can be very frustrating.
- Short-term memory problems can cause the person to forget what they have said or done and repeat themselves.
- Pain is under-diagnosed and under-treated in people with dementia, who may communicate pain non-verbally by shouting or hitting out.

These problems then have consequences for the person themselves, others who live with them and the relationships between them. For every problem, there will be an explanation linked to the condition or people's responses to it, and knowing this can help others recognise that difficulties are not caused deliberately nor are they the fault of the person with dementia. Often, adjustments to the physical environment, ways of communication or taking a problem-solving approach can enable the person to reduce or stop behaviour which others find difficult or which harms the person with dementia. An 'ABC' (Antecedent, Behaviour, Consequence) chart can reveal patterns and triggers (Table 19.1).

Common problems

Low mood

Low mood in people with dementia may be caused by the reduction in neurotransmitters associated with the condition, the person's emotional response to loss, the isolation and stigma that can co-occur or a combination of factors. Vascular dementia is associated with depression and labile mood and the person may show their feelings more because of disinhibition. Sometimes a person feels abandoned because they cannot remember a loved one's recent visit. They may feel powerless or bored in an alien environment, or there may be very little that is interesting to do. The person may feel that no one knows them, they do not 'fit in' and that they cannot develop relationships or feel part of a community. The most useful responses to low mood in people with dementia are interpersonal and activity based. Unfortunately anti-depressants are not usually effective but interventions that make a difference include:

- Showing affection and warmth, while including the person
- Speaking clearly and listening to their point of view
- Getting to know the person and providing suitable activities
- Avoiding triggers and using distraction
- Enabling contact with outdoor spaces and animals
- Singing, playing music and dancing
- Providing contact with distant family, for example, by Skype or playing a taped message or video
- Offering things to look forward to

Apathy

Apathy may be caused by lack of stimulation combined with difficulties concentrating, which hamper engagement. It may also reflect low mood. Difficulties with word finding and communication can lead to 'opting out' of conversations. Alternative ways of engaging may be more successful, for example massage, music or non-verbal humour. Many people enjoy watching TV programmes or YouTube films involving slapstick humour.

Repetitive speech

Repetitive speech is caused by having forgotten saying the phrase previously, while the trigger for the speech remains or a need is still unmet. The ideal response is to act as if it is the first time every time, then address the unmet need. Distraction through change of activity can be useful. If the speech reveals an underlying emotional need, it can be useful to think creatively about how that need can be met. So if the person with dementia asks for their parent, consider how comfort or reassurance could be given. Sometimes people repetitively request to use the toilet when they have just been. The cause may be physiological or related to an infection, so this should be investigated by the GP. If the repetition seems to reflect a need for attention, then this is an unmet need. Family members may not be able to meet the level of need, but simulated presence, for example, using a doll, might help, or the person could be encouraged to befriend another lonely person.

Following a family or professional carer is a common issue if the person is unable to express feelings of insecurity or disorientation. The feelings are alleviated by keeping a familiar trusted person within sight at all times. This can be very frustrating for the person being followed, as they feel harassed and are denied privacy. Reassurance about safety, using the radio to simulate presence or having a pet or doll can help. Ensuring that attachment is broadened to include others will allow some breathing space, but colleagues and family members need to provide relief and avoid colluding with an expectation that one person can meet all needs.

Disinhibition is often the result of damage to the frontal lobe, which controls social behaviour. Some disinhibited behaviours are upsetting but not really problematic, while others can be more challenging. The person may say things out loud that previously they would have kept to themselves, or swear, or behave in ways that are socially awkward, for example, pushing into a queue. They may behave sexually in public places (Chapter 47) in which case it is best to ensure that they are in an environment where it does not matter (a private room) or there is less opportunity for the behaviour.

Aggression

Similarly if a person with dementia feels angry, frustrated or threatened they may react aggressively (Table 19.2). If possible it is best to minimise any triggers, such as noise or over-stimulation, and to consider if the person has any unmet needs that they are unable to communicate verbally, such as toothache or painful joints (Figures 19.1 and 19.2). Resistance to personal care (see Chapter 54) is a common trigger. Warm reassurance can help defuse anger, but if possible, it is best to allow the person some space and return later.

The need for a sensitive approach

Knowing the person and empathising with their experiences promote a sensitive, positive and non-judgemental approach. However, being with a person with dementia whose behaviour demands great patience can be difficult, so family and professional carers need support and education to enable them to continue to cope with creativity and good humour. Pre-empting behaviour by anticipating needs and considering alternative ways of meeting them lead to a more relaxed life for the person with dementia and satisfaction in a role well carried out for their carer.

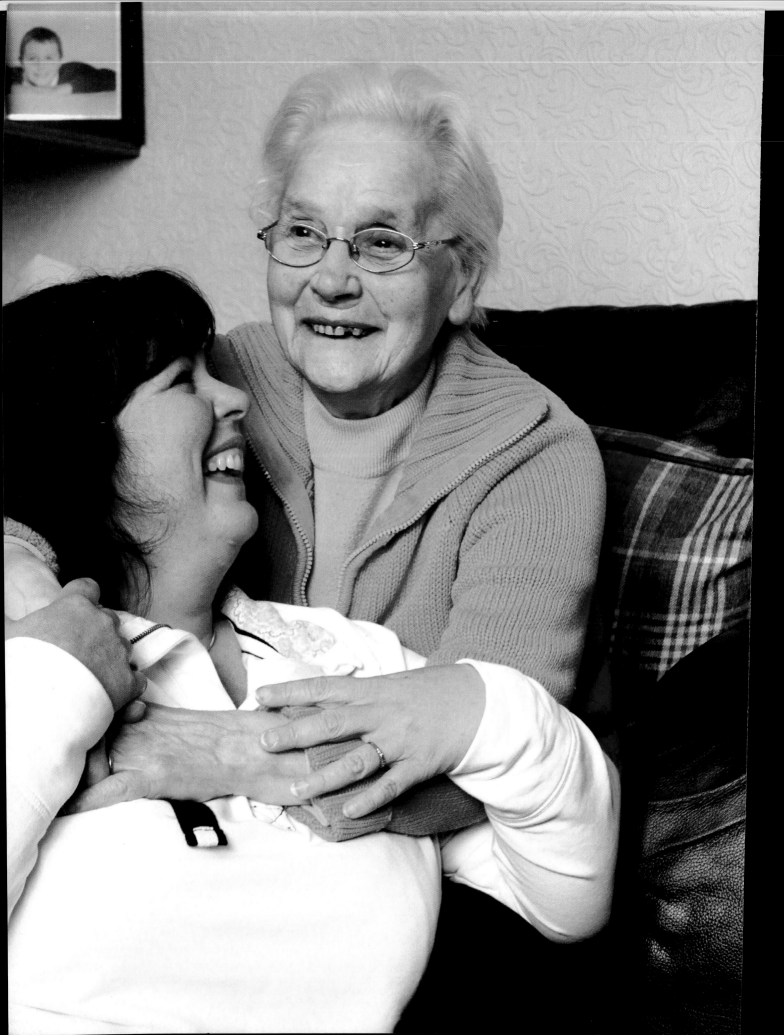

Mental health problems

Part 5

Chapters

20 Depression in people with dementia

Figure 20.1 Neurotransmitters related to depression

Acetylcholine	Opioids	Dopamine	Gamma-aminobutyric acid (GABA)	Glutamate	Serotonin	Noradrenaline
Recall and learning; in conjunction with dopamine for movement	Pain perception and modulation of pain pathways	Essential for movement; plays a role in perception of reality, motivation, reward, pleasure	The most widespread inhibitory neurotransmitter in the brain. May modulate action of noradrenaline and serotonin-releasing neurons	The most abundant excitatory neurotransmitter in the brain. May modulate cross-talk between neurons for memory formation and plays a role in neuronal death	Sleep, appetite, pain, joy	Blood pressure regulation, anxiety, motivation, focus

Mood and memory

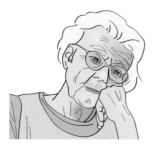

Sometimes, people explain low mood and depression in terms of chemical imbalances in the brain, but this is a somewhat simplistic approach to a complex phenomenon. Structural imaging and other studies suggest several areas of the brain – the amygdala, the thalamus, the hippocampus and the prefrontal circuits – are key circuits for mood. Communication takes place by means of multiple neurotransmitter systems in networks that enable mood, emotion and memory to emerge

Neurochemistry and depression

It is thought that projections from the key 'mood' areas influence the output of the hypothalamus, midbrain and brainstem, which organize and co-ordinate the body's physiological and behavioural responses to stressors and emotional stimuli

Table 20.1 Recognising similarities and differences between depression and dementia

Indications of low mood or depression	Indications of poor memory or dementia
Sadness	History of depression, current low mood plus disorientation
Feeling anxious	Fluctuating anxiety and agitation
Ruminative, negative thoughts	Difficulty with following logical thought processes
Tearfulness	Tearfulness, with labile (quickly changing) mood
Pessimism	Flatness, difficulty in imagining the future
Low self-esteem	Fluctuating self-esteem, increasingly poor self-awareness
Having no pleasure in life, not able to enjoy anything	Able to enjoy familiar activities and the company of others
Self-blame, guilty feeling	Sometimes accusing others, eg of taking 'lost' handbag
Difficulty remembering	Poor memory, particularly short-term
Negative, pessimistic content of conversation, slowed speech	Repetitive conversation
Self-isolation	Being left out by others
Feeling worse in the morning	Feeling worse in the afternoon or evening - 'sundowning'
Poor sleep – early morning wakening	Changes in sleep-wake cycle, disorientated in time, sleeping in the day, awake at night
Poor appetite, weight loss	Forgetting to eat, changes in food preference, weight loss
Poor concentration	Poor concentration
Low libido	Increased or decreased libido, sometimes sexual disinhibition
Lacking spontaneity in speech	Word-finding difficulty
Complaining of aches and pains	Not complaining of pain, but untreated pain results in behavioural indications of distress (crying, walking restlessly, irritable behaviour)
Constipation (due to slow metabolism and lack of food and exercise)	Constipation or incontinence, due to forgetting to go to the toilet or not recognising physiological signs of needing to go
Increased smoking or drinking more alcohol	May either smoke and drink more (having forgotten previous intake) or less

Dementia Care at a Glance, First Edition. Catharine Jenkins, Laura Ginesi and Bernie Keenan. © 2016 by John Wiley & Sons, Ltd. Published 2016 by John Wiley & Sons, Ltd.
Companion website: www.ataglanceseries.com/nursing/dementiacare

People with depression and dementia

The appearance of depression and dementia can be very similar (Table 20.1). Both conditions can make a person seem uninterested, slow to respond, not be looking after themselves properly, have poor concentration and fail to take part in life as they used to. If the person's behaviour is more dementia-related, they tend to feel worse as the day goes on. For people with depression, the early morning is usually the worst time of a day.

Causes of depression

The term 'depression' is used to cover a wide range of miserable feelings, from being briefly 'fed up' to states of feeling desperate, worthless and suicidal (Table 20.1). It is very important to assess and address persistent low mood; it can damage quality of life but can also be life-threatening. In addition, because depression and dementia have similar signs, it is possible that a person can be misdiagnosed, leading to the wrong treatment and on-going unnecessary suffering.

It is sometimes suggested that people with memory problems are unaware of what they are going through and, therefore, do not experience what might be considered a logical response to loss, that of grief or low mood. In fact, depression often does occur with dementia. Most people, at least in early stages of memory loss, are aware of their difficulty, which naturally leads to anxiety and low mood. In addition, the loss of brain cells that occurs in Alzheimer's disease leads to reduced production of the neurotransmitters such as serotonin and dopamine that are considered necessary for stable mood (Figure 20.1).

A history of depression in old age is associated with increased (about 20% higher) risk of development of dementia. While it is always important to treat low mood (with anti-depressants, talking therapy, exercise or all three), this correlation highlights the need to look after all aspects of health in building protection from dementia and maximising quality of life and well-being.

Recognising depression

Depression is a feeling of low mood, sadness and pessimism. A person with depression might have very low self-esteem and a feeling that they are useless, hopeless and getting in the way. A sensation of lacking spontaneity and something to say can lead to self-isolation. Sometimes people are tearful, but often low mood shows in ways that are less easy to decipher. Depression can lead to a sensation of lethargy, lack of energy or loss of possibility of pleasure. This sluggishness extends to physical symptoms: appetite decreases and the individual often becomes constipated, sleeps badly, any aches and pains feel worse and libido is damaged. The person takes little interest in their own appearance and that of their home; they may not look after their hygiene and wear the same clothes for days. He/she may feel there is no point to anything and show no interest in aspects of life that they used to enjoy. Very rarely, people may hallucinate and, for example, hear voices (that others cannot hear) saying horrible things to them. People may struggle to concentrate, and even when they agree that things are not right, it is difficult or impossible for them to find the motivation to change.

Other people can find it difficult to relate to a depressed person and often misinterpret their behaviour, for example, as 'laziness' or irritability. In the case of older people, depression is often mistaken for dementia, even by health professionals. Depression is a treatable condition, so if the person themselves does not have the awareness or motivation to visit their doctor, it is important that those around them support and encourage them to attend. It can be difficult to differentiate between depression and dementia, so a skilled assessment is essential.

Other peoples' responses

People with dementia describe feeling stigmatised by their diagnosis. Others do not always know how to respond and may leave the person with dementia out or ignore them. In later stages of dementia, people are sometimes talked over or made to feel incompetent. Family members and professionals should keep this in mind and make the effort to include the person by modifying their communication skills and making adjustments so that the person with dementia can be included and maintain their self-esteem. Partners of people with dementia and professionals who work with them sometimes have a similar experience of being 'stigmatised by association'. Being with someone with dementia, particularly a loved one, can be stressful, so it is important that family members and friends support carers and offer opportunities to chat and take part in group activities.

Coping with depression and low mood

Feeling in charge of one's life and that there are opportunities for fun and relating to others is good for self-esteem and mood. The person with dementia and family members can agree in advance that independence should be maintained as much as possible for the sake of the mental health of all parties. Exercise promotes optimism and people with dementia can enjoy taking part in activities they used to do, with support if necessary. Walking outdoors or round the shops (when not busy) can be enjoyable and an opportunity to exercise while meeting others. Taking part in household chores can be satisfying and reassure the person they are useful. Being involved with young people or small children often lifts mood, as relationships are non-judgemental and do not depend on complex conversation.

Unfortunately, anti-depressant medications often do not work for people with dementia. However, pain management and looking after physical health optimise well-being. The person with dementia should also be supported so that they can continue in spiritual activities. Positive friendly communication, an optimistic outlook, inclusion, activity and maintaining involvement within the community will all make a difference to mood and well-being.

21 Delirium in dementia

Box 21.1 Features of delirium

- Sudden confusion or worsening of existing confusion

- Develops suddenly over a short period, hours or days and can fluctuate throughout the day rather than at particular times

- Can be very quiet or alternatively agitated or disorientated

- Hallucinations

- Disrupted sleep patterns

- Rambling conversation or disjointed speech

- Drowsiness

- Sudden poorer short-term memory

- Reduced attention spans

- Altered mood

Box 21.2 Top tips

- Identify the condition by the sudden nature of the confusion or worsening confusion and other typical features (see Box 21.1)

- Refer to a physician for formal assessment and review

- Make sure that any underlying illness, such as infections, are treated promptly

- Be extra vigilant on the person's behalf while they have this condition, as it makes them less able to look after themselves and more at risk of injury or deteriorating health

Box 21.3 'Undertow'

Tick tock of the time piece.

Darkness slowly drains away
leaving only the ghost of the night.

Light seeps into the bedroom
revealing the dark form in the next bed.

A face, a nose, a mouth and two eyes, closed.

Grey hair spread over white.

Groping for a stick by the side of the bed
he reaches over and taps the sleeping form.

A one word response mumbled through sleepy lips.

"What's that you say?

Sleeping?

You should be ashamed,
taking advantage of an old man.

What would your employer say?

Get up and do your work!

My wife would tell you.

If she was here"

Memories drop like pebbles into a vast ocean
only to be sucked away by the undertow.

A smile, sunlight, the caress of soft skin,
black hair spread over white, blue sky.

Shadows sink to the murky depths.

The tide ebbs
leaving his sun bleached mind
adrift on the seas.

Source: *Reproduced by permission of Sue Carroll*

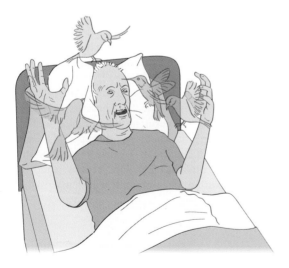

Hyperactive delirium

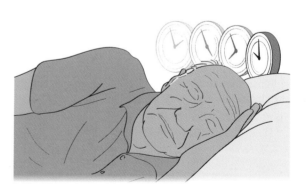

Hypoactive delirium

Dementia Care at a Glance, First Edition. Catharine Jenkins, Laura Ginesi and Bernie Keenan. © 2016 by John Wiley & Sons, Ltd. Published 2016 by John Wiley & Sons, Ltd.
Companion website: www.ataglanceseries.com/nursing/dementiacare

Definition

'Delirium' is a syndrome involving temporary or acute confusional states resulting from illness or infection. A person with delirium will have disturbed consciousness and difficulty orientating themselves to their location, the time of day and the people around. It will be difficult or impossible for them to think logically and they may be frightened by their experiences.

Although it is potentially reversible, delirium is nevertheless a serious condition causing higher death rates, increased risk of complications and longer hospital stays. In addition, it can increase the rate of functional decline in somebody with dementia. Older people are more prone to developing delirium because of reduced renal blood flow and function; they are also more likely to be taking multiple medications. Older people with dementia are estimated to have a fivefold risk of developing delirium.

Manifestations of delirium

Some of the features of delirium are described in Box 21.1 and are generally typified by a sudden confusion or worsening of existing confusion. Drowsiness and withdrawal might be observed, or alternatively increased agitation. The person may be seeing things that are not there (hallucinating) and may have rambling or disjointed speech. Short-term memory is often poorer, mood may be altered and the attention span is reduced. Typically, the disorientation or increased disorientation will have developed quickly over a matter of hours or days rather than months and may fluctuate throughout the day rather than having an observable pattern (although sleep is often disturbed). Any unusual behaviour that is out of character and of a sudden onset could be caused by delirium. Delirium can be a life-threatening illness if it is not recognised and the underlying causes treated promptly.

Causes of delirium

Delirium can be caused by any infection or illness, but chest infections and urinary tract infections are common culprits. Pathophysiology of delirium is rather poorly understood, but it is common to come across dysfunction of the stress response and exaggerated inflammatory states in elderly people; in people with dementia, these are thought to interact to induce delirium. It may be that systemic inflammation could be acting as a stressor that can trigger an acute exacerbation of the dementia. Trauma can also cause delirium, for example, fractured bones or the trauma of invasive procedures such as urinary catheterisation. The risk of delirium is particularly high in the first 48 hours after surgery with general anaesthetic. Delirium can also be triggered by dehydration, malnutrition, constipation or pain. Some medications can cause delirium, particularly if the person is taking four or more each day (multiple medications or 'polypharmacy') or if they are taking sedative preparations or medication for epilepsy.

Prevention

It is possible to reduce the likelihood of delirium occurring and promote a quicker recovery if it does occur.

Strategies to prevent delirium include:

- Encouraging regular drinks and meals
- Keeping the person active and mobile
- Offering warm milk or herbal tea instead of sleeping tablets
- Keeping medication to a minimum
- Making sure that hearing aids and spectacles are worn
- Keeping background noise to a minimum
- Not using urinary catheters
- Not using bed rails or anything that restricts movement
- Using personal objects to make surroundings more familiar
- Frequent explanations of everything that is going on
- Avoiding any unnecessary changes of location
- Treating any pain
- Encouraging family members or people with familiar faces to spend time with the person

Management Strategies

Recognising the delirium for what it is and finding the underlying cause is vital in treating the condition (Box 21.2). Consequently, referral to a physician or health professional is essential in order that a formal assessment can be made using a recognised tool, such as the Confusion Assessment Method (CAM; Inouye et al., 1990) which differentiates delirium from other causes of confusion. A medication review and routine screening for infection are also recommended. Obvious signs of infection might include temperature above 37.5C, painful urination, offensive or cloudy urine, or a rattly cough. Addressing underlying problems such as pain, dehydration, malnutrition and constipation will help.

It is important to deal with the effects of worsening disorientation; for example, more frequent orientation and reorientation may be needed at regular intervals throughout the day. A calm and reassuring approach will help enormously, as delirium is a frightening condition to experience. It is even more important for the person to have continuity of care, with the same familiar carer looking after them rather than a series of unknown faces. Carers will also have to be more vigilant on the person's behalf, as they are less able to manage independently while they suffer from this condition and, for example, are more likely to fall or become dehydrated or malnourished. Increasing supervision during this time and ensuring the person with delirium is safe, using aids such as spectacles, hearing aids or walking frames will contribute to maintaining orientation and exercise, so promoting recovery.

Excessive drowsiness

If the person with dementia is very sleepy in the day time, it can be tempting for carers to be relieved that they are resting. However, this extra sleepiness can be a sign of delirium, so it is important to monitor its extent and to encourage the person (even without delirium) to be more active in the day time so that they re-establish a healthy sleep pattern. If the person is difficult to rouse, this could be an indication of a serious problem, so medical advice should be sought.

Psychosis in people with dementia

Figure 22.1   Psychosis

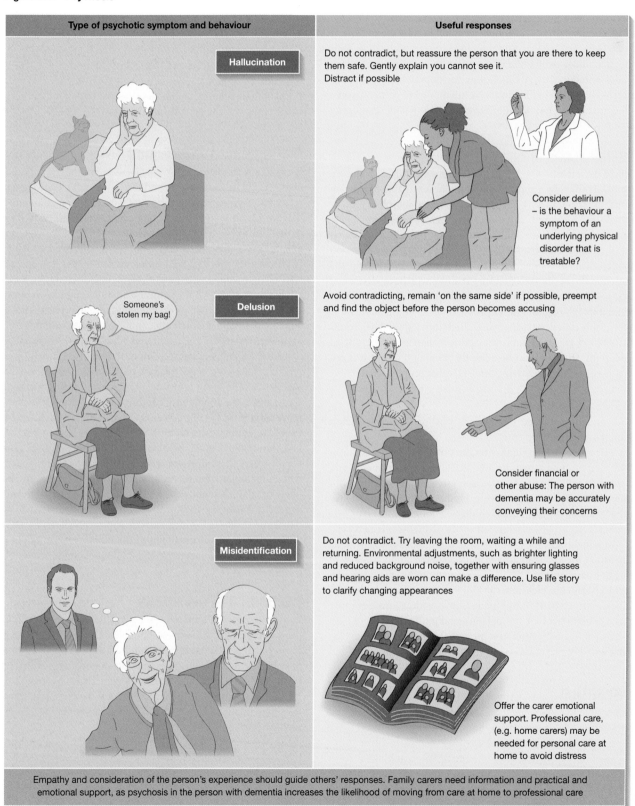

Type of psychotic symptom and behaviour	Useful responses
Hallucination	Do not contradict, but reassure the person that you are there to keep them safe. Gently explain you cannot see it. Distract if possible Consider delirium – is the behaviour a symptom of an underlying physical disorder that is treatable?
Delusion Someone's stolen my bag!	Avoid contradicting, remain 'on the same side' if possible, preempt and find the object before the person becomes accusing Consider financial or other abuse: The person with dementia may be accurately conveying their concerns
Misidentification	Do not contradict. Try leaving the room, waiting a while and returning. Environmental adjustments, such as brighter lighting and reduced background noise, together with ensuring glasses and hearing aids are worn can make a difference. Use life story to clarify changing appearances Offer the carer emotional support. Professional care, (e.g. home carers) may be needed for personal care at home to avoid distress

Empathy and consideration of the person's experience should guide others' responses. Family carers need information and practical and emotional support, as psychosis in the person with dementia increases the likelihood of moving from care at home to professional care

Dementia Care at a Glance, First Edition. Catharine Jenkins, Laura Ginesi and Bernie Keenan. © 2016 by John Wiley & Sons, Ltd. Published 2016 by John Wiley & Sons, Ltd.
Companion website: www.ataglanceseries.com/nursing/dementiacare

Defining psychosis

The term 'psychosis' refers to an experience of losing touch with reality due to symptoms such as hallucinations, delusions and disordered thinking (Figure 22.1). A hallucination involves hearing, seeing, smelling, tasting or feeling something that other people cannot. Auditory and visual hallucinations are the most common, and nothing real or obvious triggers the sight or sound that the person describes seeing or hearing. Nevertheless, the unusual thoughts and disordered thinking are very real to the person who experiences them. A delusion is a belief that has no apparent relationship with the reality perceived by others who are around the person. Delusional beliefs are usually very strongly held and immune to attempts by other people to prove them false. Unfortunately, there is a stigma linked to the serious mental health problems (e.g. schizophrenia) that are usually associated with psychosis, and many believe psychosis leads to dangerousness. Actually, people with serious mental health problems are more often a risk to themselves than other people, but (in a similar way to dementia) the stigma and exclusion that follow can be as damaging as the original issues. True psychosis is rare in dementia, and if it occurs, tends to happen in later stages. Psychosis is not easy for the person with dementia or their family members to cope with, but understanding that the person is unwell and not being deliberately difficult can make it easier to manage.

Delirium (see Chapter 21)

Sudden onset of visual and other types of hallucinations indicate a serious underlying physical condition, so a thorough assessment by a health professional should be arranged promptly. The person who is hallucinating may raise their hands and make grasping movements or follow visions with their eyes. They might mention an animal, such as a cat, on the bed. Treatment should address the cause, which is often infection or constipation.

Hallucinations and delusions in dementia

Knowing the person and their recent routine will usually enable others to detect the reason or trigger for their behaviour. In the later stages of dementia, old memories are more real than current events. A person with dementia may mention seeing someone from the past but actually could be describing a memory. The person with dementia may say they have heard someone when that person is not there. They may be communicating that they want to talk about a person who has died. Sometimes hearing aids magnify all sounds to the extent that it is difficult to tell the difference between background noises, such as TV and actual relevant conversations. Family members may sound very similar to each other, so the person with dementia may be mistaken about who they have heard. A visual hallucination (seeing something that is not there) could be caused by damaged visuoperceptual functioning (or not wearing spectacles) and originate from a shadow or a reflection, or again an old memory. Sometimes when the person forgets a word, they use a replacement with similar sound or meaning – leaving others believing that they are describing a hallucination when not the case.

Delusional beliefs are common in dementia but can usually be explained by the difficulties caused by forgetfulness. The term 'confabulation' refers to how a person with dementia makes up a likely story to fill a gap in their memory, based on either a false memory or their usual previous practice. For example, if asked what they had for breakfast, they might reply confidently 'a lovely bowl of porridge'. Although the answer would not be true, the person with dementia would not be lying as they themselves believe the answer.

If a person mislays something yet believes they are organised, it is logical to suspect that someone else has taken it. Beliefs that lead to unsubstantiated accusations can be very difficult for caring relatives to cope with, especially as professionals respond seriously in looking into concerns about adults at risk. If the person with dementia forgets that they had visitors, it is understandable that they feel low due to loneliness or thinking no one cares about them. Similarly, people with dementia may complain that they have not been fed.

Misidentification

Misidentification happens when the person with dementia does not believe the identity of a loved one, occasionally feeling that they are an imposter (Capgras syndrome) or a person from the previous generation (e.g. a daughter taken for a sister). This can be emotionally and practically very difficult, particularly when a spouse is involved. The person with dementia may miss the person they love but be remembering them as they were years ago. The older version of the relative may seem uncannily similar but may be perceived as a malicious deception. This false belief leads to fear, anger and rejection, making personal care particularly difficult. People with dementia may perceive the likeness of their own mother or father in the mirror (forgetting their own advanced age) and comment that the parent is in the house. A disorientated person in a luxurious care home may tell others they are on a cruise.

Disordered thinking

Disordered thinking can occur in later stages of dementia, as by the end of the sentence the person struggles to remember the beginning, while also forgetting names of people and objects (Chapter 18). It becomes increasingly difficult for people who are living with dementia to present ideas logically and weakened self-expression can be mistaken for delusions.

Lewy body disease

Lewy body disease can cause visual hallucinations, which are not usually frightening for the person themselves but often worry family members (Chapter 7). Anti-psychotic medications should be avoided if at all possible because of the severe risks associated with their side effects in people with this condition.

Coping strategies

Strategies like looking beneath the delusionary belief to the feeling or circumstance that triggered it and attempting to address this can help. For example, offering frequent small snacks, keeping a diary record of visitors, being more affectionate or just reminding the person with dementia where their belongings are located if they look worried.

Care and treatments

If the person with dementia seems to be frightened, they should be reassured and the cause of the hallucination or delusion removed. A thorough holistic assessment should be sought so that all possible contributing factors can be addressed. As a last resort, a small dose of anti-psychotic medication (e.g. risperidone) could be prescribed.

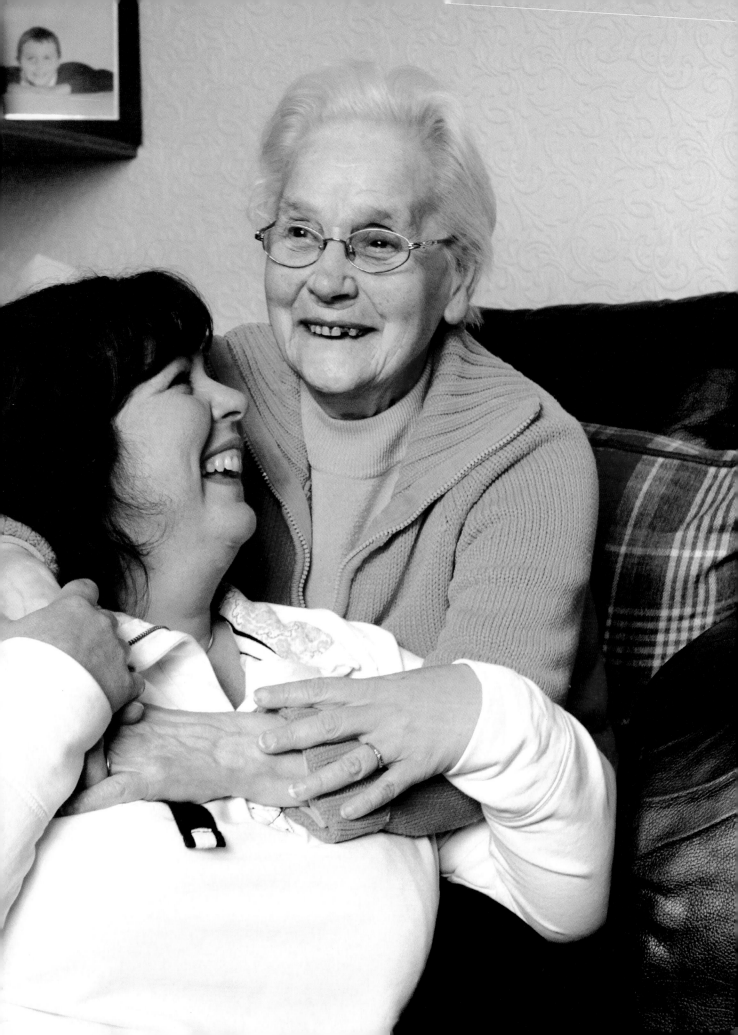

Physical health problems

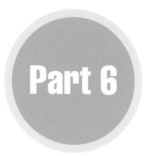

Part 6

Chapters

23 Sensory Impairment

Figure 23.1 Correct insertion of standard hearing aids (a and b) and open fit hearing aids (c and d)

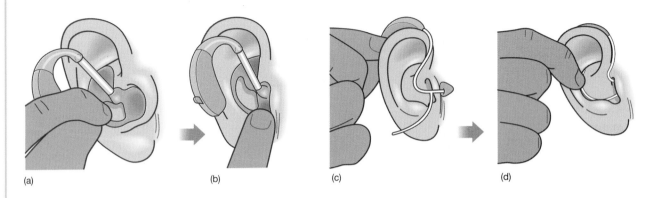

(a)   (b)   (c)   (d)

Figure 23.2 The Hospital Communication Book

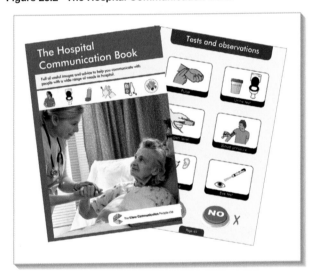

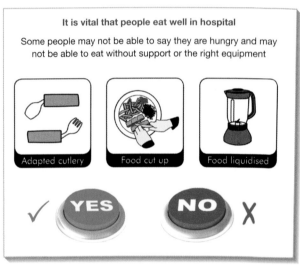

Source: *Reproduced with permission of The Clear Communication People Ltd.*

Box 23.1 Top tips

- As organs age, sensory impairments become more common; for people with dementia, sensory impairments can exacerbate any communication problems that already exist

- Annual routine tests of vision and hearing should be completed and referrals made for further assessment if problems are found

- Hearing aids and spectacles should be checked to ensure they are effective. However, getting used to new aids can be difficult for people with dementia

- Useful communication strategies include promoting lip-reading, use of gesture and touch, large print, reducing background noise and increasing light levels

- Stronger flavours can lead to increased enjoyment of food

Dementia Care at a Glance, First Edition. Catharine Jenkins, Laura Ginesi and Bernie Keenan. © 2016 by John Wiley & Sons, Ltd. Published 2016 by John Wiley & Sons, Ltd.
Companion website: www.ataglanceseries.com/nursing/dementiacare

Dementia and sensory loss

The ageing process affects sensory organs, resulting in impairment for many older people. For example, hearing loss affects 50% of people over the age of 60 years. Most older people are able to manage effectively despite some problems with their vision, hearing, taste, smell, balance and/or sense of touch. The combination of any of these difficulties with dementia adds to the disabling impact, with risk of subsequent low mood and social isolation.

Visual problems

In older age, existing visual problems or low vision tend to worsen and individuals are more likely to experience additional problems with distance and night vision. The most serious visual problems, all of which may lead to blindness, are:

- Age-related macular degeneration: A disorder of the macula section of the eye that results in loss of central vision; it is classified as dry or wet. Although there is no available treatment for the dry type, wet macular degeneration can be treated with medication to slow the progression of sight loss.
- Cataracts are opacity of the lens due to the degeneration of the lens fibres, which reduces the amount of light able to reach the retina; they can be treated by surgical removal or lens replacement.
- Glaucoma is a condition where damage to the optic nerve is caused by high intra-ocular pressure (pressure within the eye itself); it can be treated with eye drops and surgery.
- Diabetic retinopathy involves microvascular leakage or haemorrhaging in the blood vessels of the retina; it is less likely if diabetes is well controlled.

Interventions

Interventions should take into account the difficulty a person with dementia may have in adjusting to new resources and learning new skills. Opticians should be informed of the person's memory problems so that they can adjust their assessments as required. Vision tests are best scheduled for the time of day when the person with dementia is at their optimum level of functioning – this is usually the morning. Interventions include:

- Annual routine eye tests and specialist assessment of vision if any problems are identified
- Supporting and orientating the person so that they can maintain their independence
- Making sure that they are wearing their spectacles, using their magnifiers, etc. (but contact lenses pose risks for those with cognitive impairments)
- Referral to low vision support services (via GP or social services)
- Ensuring rooms are brightly lit
- Using highly delineated colour contrasts to aid orientation
- Using adapted crockery and cutlery, such as subdivided plates with deep ridges, easy grip-padded cutlery, non-slip plate mats
- Using large signage and large font size in any written material
- Specialist large-dialled phones and remote controls
- Using guide rails and careful positioning of furniture, aids and adaptations. Furniture and décor within the home environment should be kept the same, to aid orientation using long-term memory
- Providing extra night lighting
- Placing objects within the person's visual field
- Telling the person when you are present or are leaving

Hearing problems and treatments

Temporary hearing loss can be caused by a build-up of wax in the ears, which can be resolved by ear drops or/and syringing.

A middle ear infection (otitis media) will also cause temporary deafness and usually clears up without treatment within 3 days; however, if it persists it requires treatment with antibiotics. Permanent deafness can be caused by 'presbycusis', a degeneration of the sensory cells in the ear, which leaves the auditory system less sensitive to certain frequencies of sound; this cannot be reversed and a hearing aid may be required. Otosclerosis is a calcification of the joint at the stapes, which attaches to the cochlea; it can be managed by surgery or bilateral hearing aids. Tinnitus or ringing in the ears is also common; distraction and reassurance can help the person cope.

Interventions

Any hearing problems should be investigated and the cause of the deafness identified. It can be difficult for anyone to adjust to wearing a hearing aid, and separating the sounds of speech from distracting background noise can be particularly difficult for people with dementia who will need support during the adjustment process.

- Refer to specialist hearing services where appropriate (via GP).
- Annual hearing assessments should be completed.
- Make sure that any hearing aids are worn and check to see if the hearing aid is fitted into the ear properly (see Figure 23.1), that it is turned on, that the battery does not require changing and that the tube is not blocked by condensation or wax.
- Use handheld amplifiers where available.
- Get the person's attention before speaking, for example, touch the arm.
- Speak slowly and clearly using short sentences.
- Sit or stand nearer to the person, at the same height in a face-to-face position in front of the person to make lip reading easier.
- Use non-verbal cues.
- Use written information in large font size and visual aids, such as the hospital communication booklet (see Figure 23.2).
- Rephrase and check understanding where necessary.
- Limit background noise.
- Assess the safety issues associated with the hearing impairment.

Taste and smell: olfactory impairments

A poor sense of smell is associated with subsequent development of dementia. Not being able to smell can lead to problems in telling whether food is 'off' and in recognising a gas leak. While the sense of taste is usually less affected, people with dementia often gradually come to prefer stronger tastes and may choose to take more sugar in drinks and more salt on their food. 'Umami' flavouring is an alternative that can add taste to bland savoury foods and stimulate eating. People with dementia sometimes develop a taste for curries or other strongly flavoured foods that they previously avoided.

Touch

Loss of sensitivity can lead to some reduction in pain awareness and may contribute to mobility and balance difficulties.

Proprioception (or 'position sense')

The sense of where the body is in space is dependent on feedback from the other senses and from joints and muscles. This information is processed in the cerebellum. The combination of dementia-related damage to this area of the brain with sensory impairment can lead to difficulty with gait, body movement and possible falls (Chapter 24).

24 Falls

Figure 24.1   Physiological factors that may contribute to risk of falls

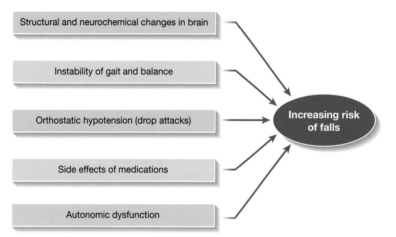

Structural and neurochemical changes in brain

Instability of gait and balance

Orthostatic hypotension (drop attacks)

Side effects of medications

Autonomic dysfunction

Increasing risk of falls

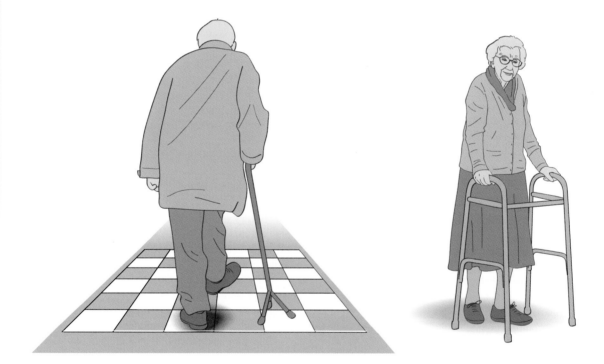

Box 24.1   Top tips

- If a person is known to fall then they should always wear supportive shoes with a good grip and have their walking aid to hand

- The person should wear any aids such as hearing aid and spectacles

- Sedation should be avoided if possible as it increases the risk of falls

- A formal falls risk assessment is essential in order to obtain the best help

- Activity (e.g. yoga, tai chi or dancing) should be encouraged to improve strength and balance

Dementia Care at a Glance, First Edition. Catharine Jenkins, Laura Ginesi and Bernie Keenan. © 2016 by John Wiley & Sons, Ltd. Published 2016 by John Wiley & Sons, Ltd.
Companion website: www.ataglanceseries.com/nursing/dementiacare

Encouraging walking and exercise is an important aspect of maintaining a person's independence and dignity, particularly for older people. More activity helps increase overall levels of fitness and is good for all the muscles – including the heart (and specifically when it involves an element of balance is associated with reduced risk of falls). However, the occurrence of falls does increase with older age and is of greater risk for somebody with dementia because they are more likely to be disorientated and perhaps unsteady on their feet, particularly if their dementia is associated with cardiovascular disease or Parkinson's disease. Older people are also more prone to suffer a fracture if they fall than would be a younger person because of increased risk of diminished bone density (osteoporosis).

Possible reasons for falls

- Poor eyesight and other visual problems
- Balance problems caused by underlying conditions such as arthritis, Parkinson's disease or previous 'strokes' (Chapter 6)
- Perceptual difficulties
- Sedation, or even just being on four or more medications simultaneously (which is common for older people)
- Long term side effects of anti-psychotic or anti-hypertensive medication
- Dizziness or vertigo caused by a variety of illnesses and conditions. These can include cardiovascular problems such as postural hypotension (also known as 'drop attacks'), where the blood pressure drops when somebody stands up suddenly (see Figure 24.1)
- Poor lighting and unsuitable/unstable furniture and flooring such as a wet or slippery surface
- Tripping over an item or pet
- Badly fitting or loose footwear
- Incontinence, as rushing to the toilet can often cause a fall
- Alcohol excess

Specialist falls services

If the older person with dementia is having falls, it is really important for them to have a formal risk assessment by a carer or healthcare professional, and for the GP or doctor in the emergency department to refer to a falls specialist and falls clinic. It is recognised that a range of interventions from such a specialist service can reduce the incidence of falls and keep the person with dementia safely independent for longer. For example, if the person is unsteady on their feet, they can be assessed for suitable footwear and walking aids to help minimise the effects of this. A cardiovascular, alcohol and medication review will be undertaken by them to exclude and address these factors as possible causes of falls. The person with dementia may not be able to avoid obvious hazards because of difficulties with visuospatial functioning (Chapter 23) and other factors such as poor eyesight, but a home assessment by a member of the falls team might identify rectifiable issues that affect safety, such as lighting or furniture placement, unsuitable/uneven flooring. The team can also offer a range of strategies to overcome the fear of falling; a recognised syndrome that often affects the person who has suffered a fall. These include not only appropriate counselling but also practical interventions, such as teaching the person how to get back up off the floor after a fall, the provision of alarms that can be worn around the neck to summon help, and a range of exercise classes to improve mobility and balance. The team will also screen for osteoporosis (thinning of the bone due to ageing), which increases the risk of serious injury following a fall and can offer mineral and vitamin supplements to help combat the effects of this.

Design and technology

Good design can make a difference; as the person with dementia may not be able to adapt to the given environment, their surroundings should be adapted to them as far as is possible. Older people with dementia are more likely to have not only the visual impairments associated with increased age but also an impaired ability to recognise objects and avoid hazards. Night vision is usually particularly badly affected. Consequently, people require increased lighting and careful use of contrasting colour and tone, for example, chequered or visually 'discordant' flooring is more likely to cause somebody with dementia to lose their balance.

Assistive technology is also available, for example, movement-activated lighting, such as floor sensors, can help avoid falls if the person gets up to walk about during the night (Chapter 44). Alarms can alert carers to the person with dementia moving but there are negative consequences of using such devices, for example chair alarms can restrict the person's mobility and make them more prone to pressure sores and loss of function. Alarm pendants worn around the persons neck can be useful in summoning assistance if they do fall, but only if they are worn, and unfortunately a person with dementia who is living on their own may forget to do this. Under-floor heating can help prevent hypothermia if an older person falls and is on the floor for a long time. A low profiling (fully lowering) bed can minimise the injuries from falling out of bed, but bed rails increase the severity of injuries, so they should only be used after a formal assessment. Simple measures can also be very effective, for example, in care settings having a traffic light system of stickers on walking frames, to denote the level of assistance and supervision required; green for fully independent with the walking aid, yellow for somebody who has some risk of falls if not supervised or guided by a carer, red for somebody who is at high risk of falls and requires constant supervision and help from one or two people.

25 Nutrition

Fig 25.1 Giving mealtime assistance

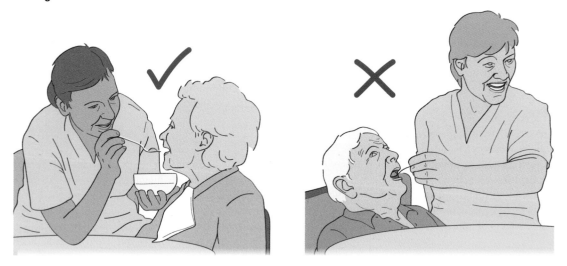

Table 25.1 Signs of malnutrition and dehydration

Poor nutritional status	Dehydration
• Progressive rapid weight loss	• Dry, cracked mouth
• Increased frailty	• Increased confusion
• Skin fragility	• Very limited urine output
• Falls	• Very dark urine
• Ketosis – breath smells like pear drops	• Sunken eyes with dark circles
• No interest in food	In extreme cases: signs of circulatory shock, e.g. thready pulse, low blood pressure, pallor
• Refusal to eat	
• On admission to care – a voracious appetite may highlight previous level of difficulty	

Figure 25.2 Enjoying a nice meal is part of everyday life and important to well-being, not just to people living with dementia. A full nutritional assessment is likely to include the following aspects:

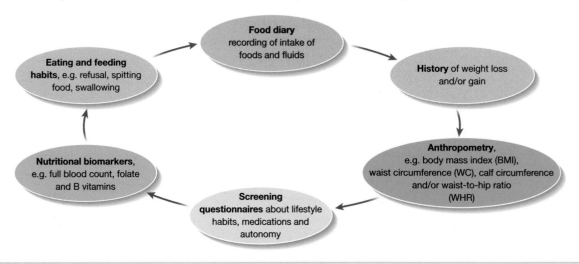

Dementia Care at a Glance, First Edition. Catharine Jenkins, Laura Ginesi and Bernie Keenan. © 2016 by John Wiley & Sons, Ltd. Published 2016 by John Wiley & Sons, Ltd.
Companion website: www.ataglanceseries.com/nursing/dementiacare

The pleasures of eating

People with dementia are usually able to enjoy food much as other people. Food that is nicely presented, with a variety of colours on the plate and is recognisably edible, is generally very welcome. Sometimes people's palates change and they may prefer food with more intense flavours (e.g. sweet or spicy) than before. Mealtimes that are sociable, with tables laid and cues that the environment is for dining all help stimulate the appetite and increase the pleasure of eating. A healthy diet not only lifts the spirits and contributes to overall well-being but also promotes better sleep, gives energy for movement and improves bowel health.

Poor nutrition in people with dementia

Under-nutrition is the result of lack of balance between intake of nutrients and energy and the body's needs and expenditure. Sometimes it arises from an inadequate diet, but alterations in digestive processes and metabolism can also contribute. Under-nutrition is common in people with dementia who may experience an earlier and more significant loss of weight in older age. Possibly, dementia-related brain shrinkage (atrophy) affects parts of the brain which are critical for regulation of appetite and energy (Chapter 3). However, cognitive factors also influence decisions about dietary intake including taste and flavour, preferences about food, availability and skills for preparation of meals; damage to the brain can affect any of these at different stages of dementia.

Achieving good nutrition for people with dementia can be difficult, for the following reasons:

- The person may not always remember to eat or recognise the feeling of hunger.
- Sometimes people do not recognise food, particularly if it is in an unfamiliar form (e.g. pureed).
- People with dementia who live alone may eat the same simple meal every day, without realising it has been some time since they had something different.
- Other people may not recognise the problem, as the person themselves will feel they are eating well and convince others this is the case.
- It may be difficult for someone with dementia to manage shopping and handling money.
- Sometimes people deliberately drink less so as to minimise toilet visits or to prevent night-time incontinence. This can lead to dehydration, constipation and reduced appetite.
- In later stages, people may have swallowing difficulties.
- Dental pain may prevent chewing, but the person may not be able to express their discomfort verbally.
- If a person needs help to eat, they need the assistance of a patient sensitive person with time to devote to the meal.
- An older person with dementia who is living on a basic state pension may not be able to afford a well-balanced diet.

Strategies to address poor nutrition

Laying the table together can help cue the person in to meal time. Family members will usually be experts in the person's food habits, for example, preferences and timing of meals. If the person needs feeding then they are much more likely to accept this from a loved one and will generally eat more. Gentle prompting and conversation during the meal can also help, but carers should be careful not to ask questions while the person is actually eating, as responding could make them gag or choke because of swallowing difficulties.

Simple environmental adaptations can help; a plate in a different colour from the table will help someone with poor eyesight to recognise it. Adapted cutlery can also help anyone with dexterity issues. Supporting the person to wear their spectacles and dentures enables them to see the food and chew it. Assistive technology (Chapter 44) can promote kitchen safety and may help the person manage at home for longer, for example, a gadget to turn the heat off on the hob if forgotten.

Assistance with eating

A person who likes to walk and finds it difficult to sit down for a length of time may need 'finger food' such as sandwiches. Someone who is not able to eat a full meal may manage smaller amounts. Those with this issue are also more likely to sit down for a drink if a carer also sits down and drinks with them, and matching movements can be helpful, as the person gradually emulates the carer in lifting the cup to their mouth. If the person with dementia needs to be fed, then the person assisting should aim to make the meal enjoyable (Figure 25.1) by smiling, talking positively about the tastiness of the food and showing appreciation of its smell. The person should be assisted to sit upright, and the person feeding them should be at the same height, at a right angle to them. Eye contact should be maintained with the person being fed, and clear simple explanations given. Small amounts of food should be placed at the front of the mouth; if too far back, the person may gag. He/she may need gentle reminders to chew or swallow if they are in the latter stages of dementia, as they gradually lose their automatic recognition and responses to food. It is important to allow sufficient time for swallowing between mouthfuls to avoid the risk of choking or vomiting. However, nutritional support, including artificial (tube) feeding, may be considered if the problem is thought to be temporary.

Malnutrition

The most obvious sign of malnutrition is significant weight loss. A malnourished person may also be tired, sluggish, low in mood and have poor concentration (Table 25.1). Poor appetite and consequent malnutrition may be a symptom of either or both dementia and depression (Chapter 20), which can be assessed for and treated. Interventions to address malnutrition include:

- Dehydration can be immediately life-threatening and requires an urgent response. Carers should assist the person to drink a glassful of water every hour and obtain medical assistance in case there is a need for intravenous fluids (a drip) to avoid hypovolaemic shock and kidney failure.
- Referral to a health professional for a formal assessment, such as the Malnutrition Universal Screening Tool (MUST; BAPEN, 2013) (Figure 25.2)
- Use of a food diary and fluid chart to monitor actual intake.
- Weigh the person regularly to check progress.
- Using a red tray in formal care environments is a dignified way to highlight that somebody needs assistance.
- Protected meal times are often used in institutional settings to avoid ward rounds and procedures during meal times.
- Family who can help with eating should be welcomed.
- Referral to a dietician and use of food supplements.

26 Protecting and caring for skin

Figure 26.1 The European Pressure Ulcer Advisory Panel, classification system

Grade of skin damage	Grade 1	The skin is intact but has pink areas which do not turn white when pressed – this may be more difficult to see on very dark skin
	Grade 2	Loss of upper skin layers, may appear as a red shallow ulcer or liquid-filled blister
	Grade 3	The underlying fatty tissue is exposed; there may be some dead sloughy tissue also visible
	Grade 4	There is full-thickness tissue loss with exposed bone, tendon or muscle

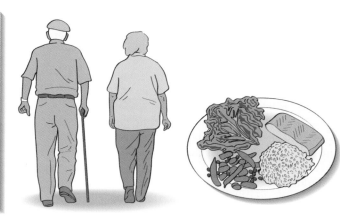

Source: *European Pressure Ulcer Advisory Panel and National Pressure Ulcer Advisory Panel (2009)*

Figure 26.2 Location and anatomy of pressure sores

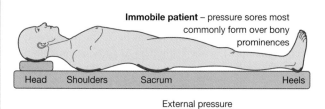

Immobile patient – pressure sores most commonly form over bony prominences

Head   Shoulders   Sacrum   Heels

External pressure (gravity/bed linen)

Bony prominence

Soft tissue

Supporting surface (e.g. mattress)

Pressure sore forms when pressure forces a bony prominence to compress the underlying soft tissue

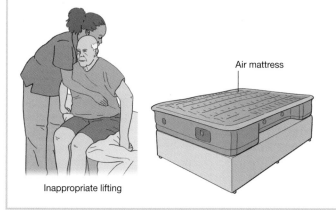

Air mattress

Inappropriate lifting

Figure 26.3 Progression of pressure sores

- The area is reddish and may be hard and warm to the touch
- Skin intact

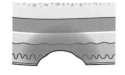

Bone — Muscle — Fat — Fascia — Skin

- Sore extends into, but not through, the skin layers
- Skin is partially lost

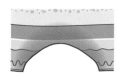

- Skin layers are completely lost
- Necrosis of subcutaneous tissue may extend to, but not through, the fascia

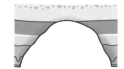

- Necrosis reaches beyond the fascia causing extensive damage to support structures, such as bone and muscle

Box 26.1 Top tips

- Keep moving, regular relief at the site of the pressure is the best way of avoiding sores
- A nutritious diet and fluids help guard the skin
- Seek specialist assessment and help as soon as possible if there is a problem
- Lifting and handling training for carers

Dementia Care at a Glance, First Edition. Catharine Jenkins, Laura Ginesi and Bernie Keenan. © 2016 by John Wiley & Sons, Ltd. Published 2016 by John Wiley & Sons, Ltd.
Companion website: www.ataglanceseries.com/nursing/dementiacare

Promoting healthy skin

Healthy skin is dependent on well-being in other aspects of a person's life. Being active, eating a healthy diet and keeping clean and dry will all contribute to healthy skin. In the early and middle stages of dementia, a person is usually able to maintain the health of their skin by eating healthily, keeping moving, washing and applying cream if necessary, either independently or with minimal help. However, in the later stages of dementia, when a person may not be so active and they may have other associated problems such as incontinence and poor mobility, skin care can become more challenging. Breaks in the skin may occur, particularly on areas that are under pressure or subject to friction (see Figure 26.2). Sometimes it is suggested that pressure sores (or pressure ulcers), are a sign of poor care. However, although good care can make a huge difference in avoiding sores or addressing pressure area care quickly, sometimes at the end of life the combination of issues such as poor nutritional and liquid intake, poor circulation, lack of mobility and incontinence can mean it is difficult to avoid skin problems completely.

Nutrition

Good nutrition and hydration is a vital element in skin health and in wound healing. Protein is essential for wound healing and muscle tone, while vitamin C and other vitamins found in fruit and vegetables support the immune system and fight infection. People with dementia are more prone to malnourishment and dehydration either because they forget to eat and drink or, as dementia progresses, they may have an impaired ability to recognise food and to swallow.

Causes of skin damage

The main causes of skin damage include:

• Pressure: where continuous pressure on skin interferes with the blood supply — this can include sitting or lying down without changing position for long periods
• Shearing: where skin is dragged or pulled against the skeleton, for example, with inappropriate lifting causing someone to be dragged up a bed.
• Friction: where a constant rubbing causes damage, for example, a badly fitted walking aid, plaster cast or oxygen piping to the nose.

The main areas where damage is likely to occur are the parts of the body where bone is most prominent and the skin is more tightly stretched over it (Figure 26.2). These can include the sacrum (bottom of the spine), buttocks, heels, elbows and the back of the head. However, any part of the body can be affected if it is exposed to direct or prolonged pressure, shearing or friction.

Particular risk factors associated with dementia

People with dementia are more at risk of skin damage for a variety of reasons. They are usually older and skin becomes thinner, drier and more prone to tearing as people age. They may not be moving around enough, and in the final stages of dementia, they may suffer a gradual loss of mobility. Alternatively, they may be actively discouraged from moving about due to fears about their safety.

As people with dementia are more likely to be dependent on others for their care, they will be dependent on their carers understanding of the need for regular movement in order to keep the skin well oxygenated and prevent tissue breakdown. They are also more likely to be incontinent, and if this is not cleaned from the skin immediately, or a barrier cream used, it will lead to tissue damage.

Strategies to avoid skin problems

Adequate levels of diet and fluids will help keep the skin healthy and guard against damage. If the skin is already damaged, then a high-protein diet (contained in milk, fish, meat and eggs) can help promote wound healing. The GP might also prescribe vitamin C and zinc supplements, which are known to assist tissue recovery. Smoking reduces vitamin C in the body and also affects the oxygenation of the skin, so it should be avoided.

Skin should be kept clean and dry at all times, and emollients used if the skin is very dry. After an episode of incontinence, the skin should be washed and all residues of soap thoroughly rinsed away, as traces of soap on the skin can also contribute to skin breakdown. The skin should be completely dried and a barrier cream used to protect the skin against the acidic moisture of urine or faeces.

Regular inspection of the skin is essential in order to detect the early stages of tissue damage (Figure 26.3) In care settings, a formal skin risk assessment chart should be completed by a health care professional, for example, the Waterlow (2005) tool. This will indicate the level of risk and what preventative measures are required.

Specialist care

If the skin is damaged, then specialist input from a district nurse will be required to dress the wound. If the damage is severe, then a referral should be made to a tissue viability specialist for expert advice, accessible via the GP or hospital depending where the person is being cared for.

Pressure area care

Moving the person to relieve the pressure is the most effective means of pressure relief, so encouraging 2–4 hourly mobilising is ideal during the day. When in bed, the person should be encouraged to change position regularly. Careful handling is required by carers in order to avoid shearing when moving someone, and all equipment should be reviewed regarding risk of friction/rubbing. If the person's ability to move is restricted, there are devices available to assist in relieving pressure.

Devices that can help relieve pressure

• Alternating air mattresses and specialist foam mattresses can be used to relieve pressure on the skin.
• Air cushions are also available for chairs, and indeed specialist chairs are available with some pressure-relieving properties inbuilt.
• Specialist products are also available for areas such as heels, elbows and nose.
• Mechanical hoists can help lift the person off affected areas when mobility is severely restricted.

27 Continence

Table 27.1 Types of incontinence

Type	Definition	Examples of causes
Stress incontinence	Involuntary leakage of urine when coughing or laughing	Damage to pelvic floor due to childbirth, or prostate problems
Urgency incontinence	A sudden urgent desire to empty the bladder, which may mean that the person cannot get there in time	Overactive bladder, urinary tract infection
Functional incontinence	Factors that cause the person to be unable to get to the toilet on time	Poor mobility, impaired vision or dexterity, cognitive problems
Overflow incontinence	When the bladder does not empty properly leading to continual dribbling	Prostate problems, constipation, nerve damage (e.g. caused by diabetes, multiple sclerosis, motor neurone disease)
Mixed urinary incontinence	Where both stress and urgency incontinence are present simultaneously	Damage to pelvic floor, damage to urethral sphincter, urinary tract infections
Faecal incontinence	Involuntary leakage of faeces	Diarrhoea, bowel disease, constipation with overflow, anal sphincter damage, neurological impairment

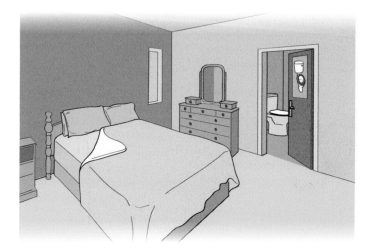

Figure 27.1 Control of the lower urinary tract, the detrusor muscle of the bladder and the micturition reflex is from the brainstem

Overactivity of the bladder muscle, leading to feelings of urgency, uninhibited bladder contractions and incontinence, may be associated with damage within the CNS, bladder irritation from infection, impaired contractility and difficulty with retention

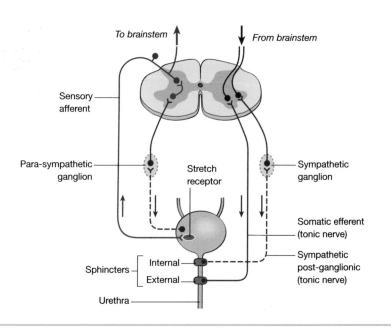

Dementia Care at a Glance, First Edition. Catharine Jenkins, Laura Ginesi and Bernie Keenan. © 2016 by John Wiley & Sons, Ltd. Published 2016 by John Wiley & Sons, Ltd.
Companion website: www.ataglanceseries.com/nursing/dementiacare

Continence

Continence is an emotive issue, as loss of control of the bladder or bowel (incontinence) has shameful connotations in our society because it is associated with child-like states or 'dirty' behaviour. It is an unpleasant and embarrassing problem to deal with, and for family members it can often be the straw that breaks the camel's back in terms of carer stress. Older people with dementia are more likely to become incontinent for a variety of reasons (see Table 27.1). Not only are they more prone to problems because of the effects of ageing, but cognitive impairment also increases the likelihood of incontinence. For example, people with dementia may be confused as to where the toilet is, or it may be that they no longer recognise it as a toilet or mistake other inappropriate objects for the toilet. They may also attempt to maintain their dignity by 'hiding' soiled clothes or urine/faeces. It is important for carers to recognise how distressing this is for the person concerned and to do all they can to maintain their privacy and dignity, as it is very easy for a person in this situation to feel dehumanised and humiliated.

Assessment

Assessing the nature of the problem can help in responding appropriately (Figure 27.1). A 3-day bladder 'diary' of how often the person is being incontinent and how much they are passing can help establish a pattern. Similarly, the use of a formal stool chart, such as the Bristol stool chart, may help in identifying different bowel problems. A full physical examination by the GP or other relevant health professional is also necessary to diagnose different bladder, urethral, uterine, pelvic floor anal sphincter or bowel problems. This may include the use of a bladder scan, which is a non-invasive procedure using ultrasound waves to check the bladder. A sample of urine should also be tested, as urinary infections can cause temporary urinary incontinence that can be easily treated with anti-bacterial medications.

Mobility

Proximity and access to the toilet are important, particularly if there are mobility issues. If the only available toilet at home is upstairs and the person cannot get there in time, then use of a commode in a private place downstairs may be an option. In a formal care setting, of course, this would not be appropriate for reasons of privacy, dignity and infection control; for example, the use of a commode behind a flimsy curtain in a multi-bedded ward area would be considered very poor practice. Having mobility aids to hand is helpful and supervising or assisting the person may be necessary, for example, wheeling them to the toilet so that they can get there in time and allowing them to walk back in order to maintain their mobility.

Behavioural management

Behavioural management can be of benefit. For example, two hourly prompted voiding of urine during the day can avoid incontinence, and extending the periods gradually can 'retrain' the bladder. Offering or suggesting the toilet following meals can also help prevent incontinence; for example, the urge to open the bowels is often triggered by a meal. In formal care settings, it is important to mimic the person's normal routines at home, as most people have optimum times when they like to have their bowels open, or empty their bladders. People with dementia may be unable to communicate their need to go to the toilet and may instead demonstrate agitation, wandering, fidgeting or pain. They may also have their own terms for the toilet or needing to use it. Involving the family in care is vital in terms of utilising their expert knowledge of the person and their usual habits and ways of expressing their needs.

Helpful design

Being within clear sight of a toilet, particularly if there is a large pictorial sign on the door, is known to improve the continence of people with dementia. Clear signage makes it easier to find the toilet and also acts as a prompt to use it. Brightly coloured or highly contrasting doors to toilets can help people to identify them more easily; similarly, a highly contrasting toilet seat can be very useful. Raised toilet seats and grab rails can be of benefit, and the toilets should be well lit, as older people are more likely to have impaired vision. People with dementia are more likely to retain their longer-term memory, so it is important to key into this by using traditional looking taps, sinks and flush handles rather than highly modern designs, which can be confusing. Easily removable clothing such as Velcro instead of zips in skirts or trousers can help people with dexterity problems like arthritis, and products such as 'helping hands' can assist with removing underpants quickly.

Diet and lifestyle

It is important to ensure that the person is not dehydrated, as they may be restricting fluids in an effort to manage their incontinence; dehydration causes the urine to become more concentrated with the consequence that urinary infections are more likely. A high-fibre diet rich in fruit and vegetables is necessary to avoid constipation, and regular exercise can help with this too (see Chapters 25 and 29). Caffeine, alcohol and nicotine can all act as bladder stimulants and should be discouraged late at night (Chapter 53). Incontinence makes the skin more prone to sores, and it is important to check the skin regularly for this (Chapter 26). If the person is incontinent they should be cleaned and dried immediately and a barrier cream should be used to prevent skin breakdown.

Specialist services

Referral to a continence specialist and continence services can help access a wide variety of resources and treatments. These can include pelvic floor exercises to strengthen the pelvic muscles, Botox injections to treat overactive urethral sphincters and medication to improve bladder tone. When all else fails, they may recommend continence products such as pads, or urinary sheaths, but these need to be checked frequently, as they can make the skin more prone to damage. Catheters may be used in palliative care situations to keep a patient comfortable when they are near the end of life. They would otherwise be a last resort for a person with dementia, as they increase trauma and the risk of infection or further damage; they also restrict mobility and impinge upon the person's dignity and expression of sexuality.

28 Constipation

Box 28.1 Signs of constipation

- Not passing a bowel motion for over 3 days

- Swollen or 'distended' abdomen

- Sudden confusion or worsening of existing confusion

- Signs of pain; wincing, rubbing abdomen, grimacing, bringing legs up to abdomen, folding arms across abdomen and huddling into a ball

- Exacerbation of agitation (which may include pacing, wandering or putting fingers into anus)

- Drowsiness, fatigue

- Poor appetite

- Headache

- Faecal overflow – when only brown liquid is coming from the anus though the person is known to be constipated

- Passing only small 'pellets' of very hard faeces

Figure 28.2 Preventing constipation

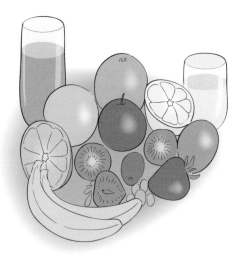

Figure 28.1 Proper toileting position

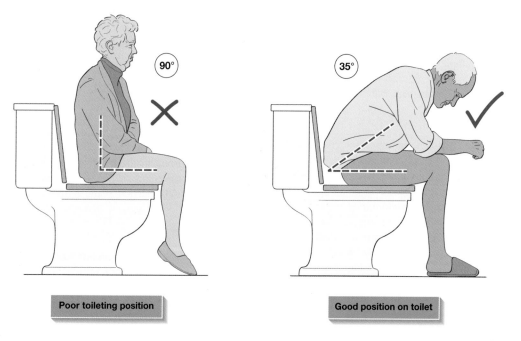

Poor toileting position

Good position on toilet

Box 28.2 Top tips

- People with dementia are more prone to constipation, particularly if they are older adults

- They may be unable to say what is wrong, so others should be vigilant for signs of constipation

- If constipation is suspected, then referral to a health professional is required for formal assessment

- Regular access to a private toilet space is probably the single most important thing we can do to avoid constipation

- Design features can act as prompts and aid recognition

- Regular exercise and a high-fibre diet can help avoid constipation

Dementia Care at a Glance, First Edition. Catharine Jenkins, Laura Ginesi and Bernie Keenan © 2016 by John Wiley & Sons, Ltd. Published 2016 by John Wiley & Sons, Ltd.
Companion website: www.ataglanceseries.com/nursing/dementiacare

Constipation

'Constipation' is a term used for difficult or infrequent passing of bowel motions. However, we all differ in our bowel habits, so a 'normal' pattern can vary from more than once a day to once every 3 days. Older people, in particular, get very concerned about having regular bowel movements, as they have often been brought up to believe that it is 'unhealthy' to miss a bowel movement, which contributes to their anxiety if this occurs. Constipation can also be very uncomfortable or even painful, and straining can exacerbate other conditions such as 'piles' (haemorrhoids), anal fissures or rectal prolapses. People with dementia may be unable to tell others that they are becoming constipated, so there is a need to be vigilant for obvious signs of this (Box 28.1).

Causes of constipation

Constipation is more common in people who have dementia, particularly if they are older adults. For example, we all have an optimum time of day when it is part of our routine to have our bowels opened, and if we are too disorientated to get there at this time, then we may lose the sensation to have our bowels opened that day. We all require privacy in order to relax and have our bowels opened, and people with dementia are more likely to be cared for in settings where privacy is not total, which may be necessary for their safety but can be inhibiting in terms of bowel movements. Eating also stimulates a bowel movement, and people with dementia are more likely to have eating difficulties or not to be eating a balanced diet with plenty of high fibre from fruit and vegetables, or even drinking sufficiently to keep the stool soft enough to pass easily.

Getting older affects the speed of metabolism, which impacts on our digestion and absorption of food. There is also impaired rectal sensation, so larger volumes are required to trigger a bowel movement. Older people are also more likely to be on medication for other conditions, and this medication can be constipatory, for example, codeine, iron and anti-cholinergics. Mobility is also affected by older age, which impacts not only on the ability to get to the toilet in time to respond to the signals to have our bowels opened, but also on the ability to get sufficient exercise to stimulate a bowel movement. We all lose physical height as we get older, which can make it difficult for the feet to be placed in the right position when seated on the toilet to tilt the pelvis and use the abdominal muscles effectively to defecate (see Figure 28.1).

Treatment of constipation

In mild cases, drinking more water, eating more fruit and vegetables and taking more exercise should help. In more serious cases, referral to a physician or health professional is essential so that a formal assessment can take place. The doctor may prescribe bulking agents or laxatives to help address the problem, but if these are not effective, then rectal stimulants such as suppositories or enemas may be required. The health professionals will also need to review the person's current medication to minimise constipatory preparations as much as possible. There is also a need to treat any conditions that make the person reluctant to have their bowels opened because of pain, such as 'piles' or rectal fissures.

Strategies to prevent constipation

Probably the single most important thing we can do to avoid constipation is to regularly encourage the person to use an accessible toilet that offers sufficient privacy to maintain their dignity and allow them to relax enough to have their bowels opened. If they have mobility issues, they may need to be helped to get there in sufficient time, and a raised toilet seat and handrails can help them to transfer onto the toilet when inside the bathroom. Large pictorials and signs will help them to recognise the room as a toilet and will act as a prompt and a highly differentiated toilet seat also helps with recognition and coordination. Mimicking normal routines in terms of timed toileting is much more likely to be successful and becoming familiar with the person's individual terms for the toilet helps us to respond to their needs promptly. If the person has problems with their feet not being able to reach the floor properly when on the toilet (particularly if a raised toilet seat is being used), then resting the feet on a small stool can help get in the best position for passing a motion; there is then a need to be careful that the person does not trip over the stool when getting on or off the toilet.

Lifestyle changes are important (Chapter 10), as, for example, obese people are more likely to suffer from constipation. Regular exercise can assist not only to maintain a healthy weight and general well-being but to also act as a stimulant to the bowels. Avoiding foods that are rich in fat and sugar can help, and encouraging a high-fibre diet that contains at least five portions of fruit or vegetables can provide the bulk people need to form adequate stools (Figure 28.2). Six to eight mugfuls of liquid per day are required to help avoid hard dried-out stools that are difficult to pass. Natural laxatives such as fruit juice or prunes are often very effective and always worth trying before resorting to pharmaceutical preparations.

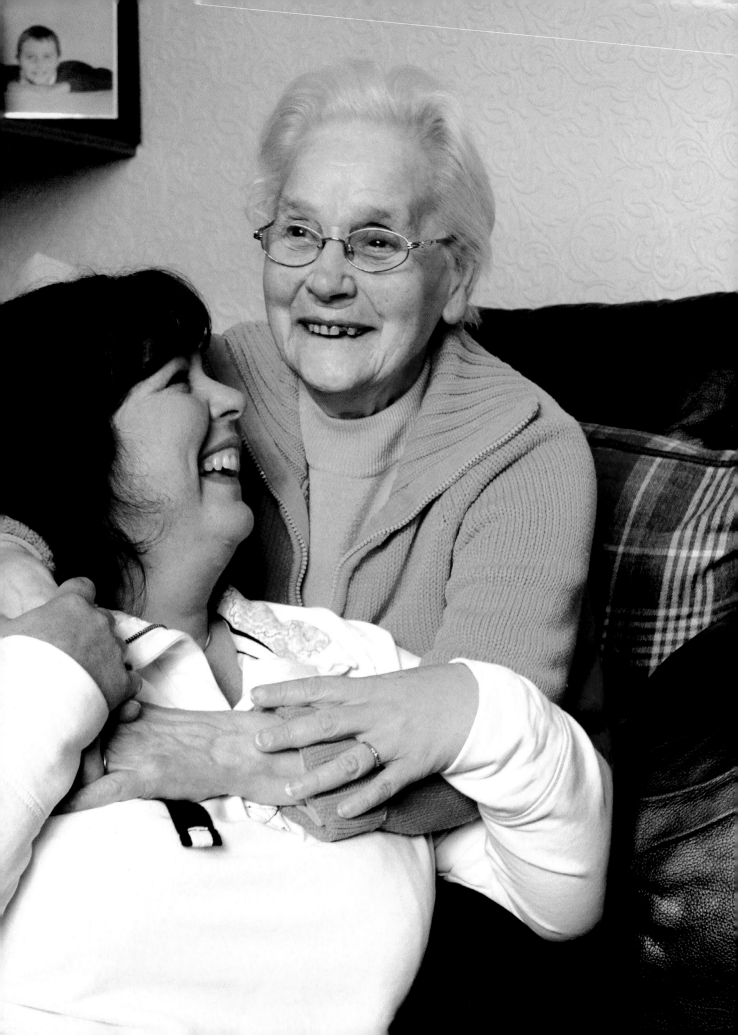

Interventions

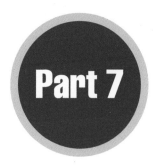

Part 7

Chapters

29 Exercise and dementia

Figure 29.1 People who exercised three or more times per week are more likely to be dementia free than those who exercised fewer than three times per week

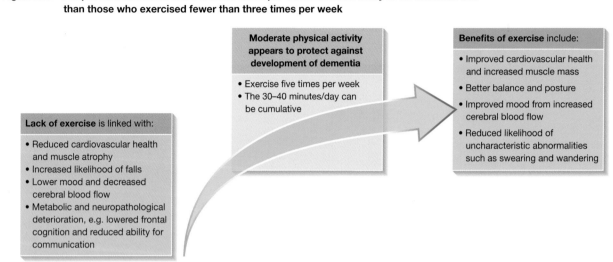

Moderate physical activity appears to protect against development of dementia

- Exercise five times per week
- The 30–40 minutes/day can be cumulative

Benefits of exercise include:

- Improved cardiovascular health and increased muscle mass
- Better balance and posture
- Improved mood from increased cerebral blood flow
- Reduced likelihood of uncharacteristic abnormalities such as swearing and wandering

Lack of exercise is linked with:

- Reduced cardiovascular health and muscle atrophy
- Increased likelihood of falls
- Lower mood and decreased cerebral blood flow
- Metabolic and neuropathological deterioration, e.g. lowered frontal cognition and reduced ability for communication

Figure 29.2 Possible physiological basis for preservation of brain function through physical activity and exercise

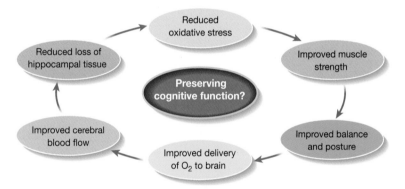

Reduced oxidative stress

Improved muscle strength

Reduced loss of hippocampal tissue

Preserving cognitive function?

Improved balance and posture

Improved cerebral blood flow

Improved delivery of O_2 to brain

Figure 29.3 Non-pharmacological approaches like dancing and yoga may be effective in slowing progression of dementia and are enjoyable for those with dementia and their carers

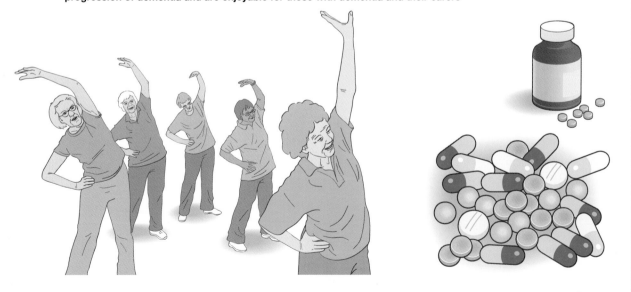

Dementia Care at a Glance, First Edition. Catharine Jenkins, Laura Ginesi and Bernie Keenan. © 2016 by John Wiley & Sons, Ltd. Published 2016 by John Wiley & Sons, Ltd.
Companion website: www.ataglanceseries.com/nursing/dementiacare

Physical inactivity and dementia

The 20th century saw the successful introduction of strategies and approaches that improved health and well-being outcomes amongst children, young people and adults, resulting in the demonstrable increase in average lifespan which is expected to affect populations for at least the coming 50 years. Since the numbers of people with dementia are expected to grow in the coming decades, it is becoming increasingly important to find potential protective factors that promote normal cognitive function into old age and prevent loss of neurons. Unfortunately, the historic trend has been based around hopes that a pharmaceutical approach for prevention and treatment of cognitive decline – a 'magic pill' – might be developed. The relentless, progressive decline in ability to undertake activities of daily living (ADL) – feeding, washing, grooming, dressing and toileting – is often one of the most alarming and troubling aspects of dementia that leads to increased dependence on caregivers and greater levels of distress. On a positive note, there is a growing body of compelling evidence from research studies that suggests that greater amounts of aerobic exercise may support cerebrovascular health and reduce risk of dementia (Figure 29.1; and see Larson and Wang (2006) in the Recommended Reading).

Later life and risk of cognitive impairment

It is clear that older people are keen to live longer and that they appreciate good quality of life just as much as everyone else. Lifestyle choice is a contributory aspect to risk factors associated with the onset of dementia, and modifiable risk factors include mid-life obesity, hypertension, diabetes, physical inactivity and depression (Chapter 10). For centuries, it has been known that exercise is an effective strategy for:

- Promoting cardiovascular health
- Improving stamina, flexibility and endurance
- Positive impacts on mood, mind and spirit
- Improved relationships with other people
- Feelings of connectedness with the environment

The complexity of pathways by which physical activity exerts its effects on brain health and neuronal plasticity has led to much debate amongst health professionals; it is difficult to isolate a single factor that is beneficial. Nevertheless, improved understanding of physiological mechanisms that contribute to poor health outcomes as a result of sedentary lifestyles can also be applied to the care of people with dementia. Knowledge of this could also be a helpful incentive for the growing number of people who are expressing awareness of dementing illnesses and their fears for their own future cognitive health.

Potential benefits of physical activity

Physical activity is any bodily activity that sustains or enhances physical fitness and well-being, and there are many reasons why people take part in physical activity. One of the most frequently mentioned benefits for people with dementia is an improvement in blood flow to the brain (cerebral perfusion), which improves oxygenation and nutrient supply (Chapter 6). Within the brain, exercise-induced changes in levels of reactive oxygen molecules may promote optimal function and neuronal cell growth.

The brain appears to retain its natural capacity for plasticity (Chapter 4) well into later life. Relatively modest amounts of physical activity seem to be sufficient to improve function and increase the size of brain areas, including the prefrontal and hippocampal areas, which may lead to reductions in memory impairments and impact on executive functions (Figure 29.2). Walking briskly for 30–40 minutes each day three times a week seems to offset the onset of dementia.

People who have dementia often lose muscle (atrophy), which can contribute to a loss of strength necessary for ADLs and an increased risk of falling (Chapter 24). Exercise strengthens muscles – they depend on being used for strength and force development – so aerobic activity can contribute to improved ambulatory status and balance.

'Walking with purpose' may meet the need for exercise and improve sleep patterns (Chapter 57).

Confidence and self-efficacy

A key aim of improving levels of exercise for people with dementia focuses on regaining time spent in unassisted ADLs, that is, improved ability to stand, walk and engage in activities with family and caregivers. It seems to be important to focus on best use of the affected person's own resources as a way of promoting self-efficacy and confidence.

The physical and psychological consequences of falling, for example, wound healing time and loss of confidence, can be considerable (Chapter 24). Bone-strengthening exercises and weight-bearing activity can help to delay the onset of osteoporosis and may be implemented as a strategy to prevent these undesirable events.

It is not unusual for people with AD or other forms of dementia to experience low mood or depression, but the beneficial effect of exercise on mood is now well established. Indeed, aerobic activities have been found to reduce the physiological response to stress and improve people's sense of well-being, probably through activation of reward and pleasure pathways in the brain.

Positive encouragement for exercising regularly and for maintaining ability to care for oneself might include small awards like 'stars' or applause. Group sessions can be a source of support when familiar caregivers are present to provide a feeling of reassurance for people with dementia; they could include Mindfulness or guided relaxation and Yoga-based breathing exercises or meditation to enable people with dementia and their familiar caregivers' to relax (Figure 29.3).

How much physical activity is beneficial?

Although further research in this area is urgently needed, moderate-intensity physical activity for 60 minutes each day is recommended. Exercise can be done to familiar music and appropriate physical activity interventions include walking, stretching, bending, dancing, lifting, Yoga-type stretches, tai chi, seated/wheelchair exercises or gardening – all use major muscle groups. Involving people in the choice of physical activity will also help to maintain a sense of energy, sheer enjoyment and fun. Healthcare providers who work with people with dementia should feel confident in encouraging participation in physical activity and exercise. Life with dementia can be difficult for everyone and it may be that taking part in exercise sessions with loved ones who have dementia could help families to cope better with caring in the home for longer, thus improving quality of life for all.

30 Dementia-friendly communities

Figure 30.1 Dementia-friendly toilet sign

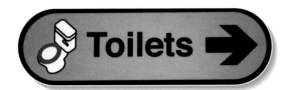

Figure 30.2 Colour can be used to highlight the shape of the toilet seat and give a 'cue'

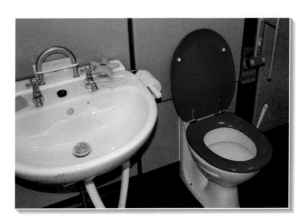

Figure 30.3 Hogewey Village for people with dementia, Holland

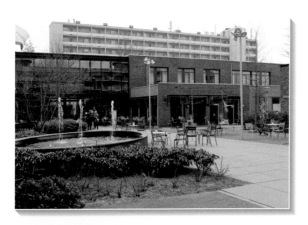

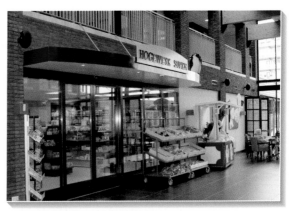

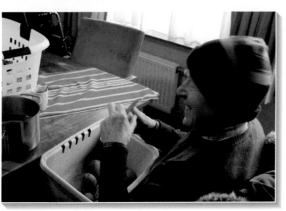

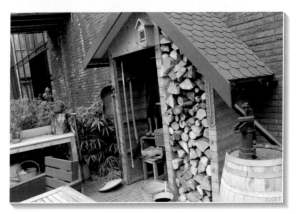

Dementia Care at a Glance, First Edition. Catharine Jenkins, Laura Ginesi and Bernie Keenan. © 2016 by John Wiley & Sons, Ltd. Published 2016 by John Wiley & Sons, Ltd.
Companion website: www.ataglanceseries.com/nursing/dementiacare

Dementia-friendliness

A community that is 'dementia-friendly' is one that welcomes the contributions of people with dementia and includes them in the network of local relationships and activities (Figure 30.3). These outcomes are achieved through a series of steps that address both the physical environment and the attitudes of people employed in local services, while promoting positivity and reducing stigma within the wider population. Most people with dementia prefer to live in their own home in a familiar location. In addition, people of all ages are gradually becoming aware of the likelihood of having a loved one with dementia, or developing it oneself. Therefore, an interest in the well-being of people with dementia within their community is about everyone's well-being.

Anyone who has been away to a foreign country and attempted to find their way around while not understanding the language or rules about traffic and pedestrians' behaviour will have some insight into some of the feelings people with dementia may experience when they are at risk of getting lost or being outpaced by the changes in their environment. Sometimes these changes and the feelings that result lead people with dementia to give up on their independent activities and remain at home, feeling lonely.

Living with dementia is an emotional and bodily experience that takes place in a social world in a geographical location. Enabling physical environments that deliberately promote independence, inter-dependence, engagement in activities and participation in supportive interpersonal relationships can maximise abilities and enjoyment of life. At the same time, public understanding of the disabilities that dementia can lead to, alongside clarity of simple adjustments (e.g. in communication skills) that can make a difference to provision of public services mean that everyone can take part in making their community dementia-friendly.

The objectives of environmental changes

The aim is to provide environments where people with dementia feel safe, are safe and are able to maintain their abilities, independence and inter-dependence so that they can live as they wish as part of a local, familiar community. Dementia causes difficulties adjusting to change, and with orientation, communication and managing sequenced steps of an activity. Therefore, buildings and spaces that have clarity of purpose, clear directions and a structure that supports calm conversation are beneficial. The environment can also promote a sense of belonging, of being welcomed and accepted, together with opportunities for activity and relaxation. In addition, as for most people, it is very important to know how to get to the nearest toilet (Figure 30.1) and to know that it will be recognisable and accessible (Figure 30.2).

The physical environment

Wayfinding

The needs of people with dementia for orientation should be considered at every stage of planning the environment. Cues are prompts that give clues and are particularly important for people with dementia who may have difficulties with orientation. Therefore, cues should be incorporated into building design so that people are aware of the purpose of the wider location and of each street and building. Changes should be made over time, when needed. So, for example, a high street's purpose could be 'readable' through:

- The appearance of the shops, banks and cafes
- A place's functions should also be clarified by its name
- Entrances should be identifiable and easy to negotiate
- Street names should be written in an easily readable font, in dark writing on a pale background, displayed in a visible location
- Signs should be used for directions, and combine words with symbols, but not confuse by having many on the same post
- Side streets should have a different appearance to the main road
- Safe places to cross the road should be recognisable, for example, by an island in the middle of the road, clear crossings and so on
- Hand rails are useful on slopes or by steps
- It is useful if there is a good view as one street leads to another, with landmarks, for example, a tree or memorial, which can become orientating cues

Design

The function of each part of the environment can be enhanced and clarified through its design, making it user-friendly. Patterns and colour changes can be confusing for people with dementia, so pathways should be defined by being a different colour from roads, while paving should be smooth and matt. Street furniture, such as communal seating, should be recognisable and stand out from the background. Mixed-generation use can be encouraged by locating seating where it will be useful for people from different sections of the community. Green space, trees and planting could promote walking and relaxation. Lighting is important, as people with dementia need more light in order to feel safe and to take in visual cues. Too many cues can be overwhelming though, so clutter and bright hoardings should be minimised.

The social environment

The social environment refers to the nature of interpersonal relationships within a group. People with dementia are sensitive to others' responses, so awareness raising, brief communication skills training and promoting commitment to the well-being of people with dementia are worthwhile. Promoting understanding of the fact that people with dementia may repeat themselves or get a little flustered is important. Learning to respond politely and patiently mean that those serving the public in shops or banks will be better able to meet the needs of their customers. People working in community organisations such as libraries and sports centres can similarly be offered basic training so that they promote social inclusion as part of their role.

Hogewey village

In Hogewey, near Weesp, in Holland, a whole village has been designed for people with advanced dementia (Figure 30.3). Here, a specific physical and social environment has been created in order to meet their needs (Jenkins and Smythe, 2013). People with dementia are supported to go about everyday life and take part in ordinary activities of daily living, cultural events and hobbies.

31 Medication for dementia-related problems

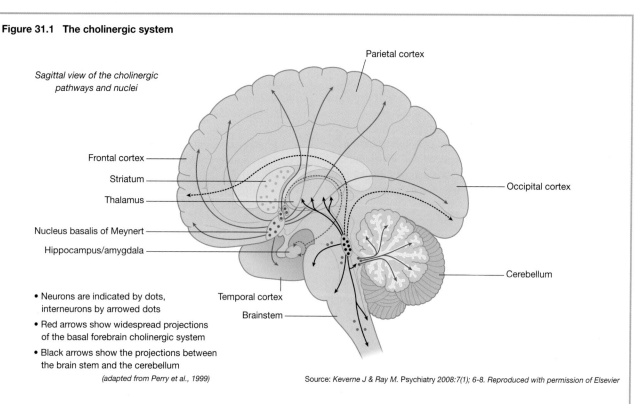

Figure 31.1 The cholinergic system

Sagittal view of the cholinergic pathways and nuclei

Parietal cortex

Frontal cortex

Striatum

Thalamus

Nucleus basalis of Meynert

Hippocampus/amygdala

Occipital cortex

Cerebellum

Temporal cortex

Brainstem

- Neurons are indicated by dots, interneurons by arrowed dots
- Red arrows show widespread projections of the basal forebrain cholinergic system
- Black arrows show the projections between the brain stem and the cerebellum

(adapted from Perry et al., 1999)

Source: *Keverne J & Ray M.* Psychiatry 2008:7(1); 6-8. *Reproduced with permission of Elsevier*

Dysfunction and loss of the cholinergic system of the neocortex is one of the earliest pathophysiological events of Alzheimer's disease.
- Acetylcholinesterase inhibitors improve cognition by increasing levels of acetylcholine
- Memantine protects neurons (including cholinergic ones) from over-exitation in response to damage

Figure 31.2 Number of people with dementia and the percentage of those receiving an antipsychotic medication prescription, time trend, (England)

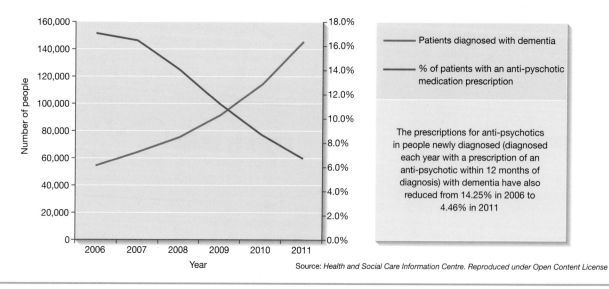

Patients diagnosed with dementia

% of patients with an anti-pyschotic medication prescription

The prescriptions for anti-psychotics in people newly diagnosed (diagnosed each year with a prescription of an anti-psychotic within 12 months of diagnosis) with dementia have also reduced from 14.25% in 2006 to 4.46% in 2011

Source: *Health and Social Care Information Centre. Reproduced under Open Content License*

There are currently no cures for dementia of any type, but there are medications available that slow progression of the conditions for some people and research is on-going in the quest for preventative and curative treatments. Dementia generally affects older people, so many will have concurrent physical health problems such as heart disease, arthritis, respiratory problems and diabetes. They may also be prone to falls (Chapter 24) and sleep problems (Chapter 55), so some people with dementia will require a variety of medications in addition to those for dementia.

Problem-solving for issues raised by dementia should focus on non-medical solutions first, with medication seen as a last resort. If essential, prescriptions should 'start low, go slow' to take account of the changing metabolism of older people, minimise adverse effects and find the smallest effective dose.

Anti-dementia drugs

The cholinesterase inhibitor medications (Chapter 32) are effective for some people with Alzheimer's disease and Lewy body disease, but are not usually effective in vascular dementia, except when it is 'mixed' with Alzheimer's. The anti-dementia drugs work for between 40% and 70% of people, delaying progression of the condition temporarily. However, the impact is positive on mood, communication and activities of daily living as well as memory, all of which make life more enjoyable for the person with dementia and are valued by family (Figure 31.1).

Anti-depressants

Depression in old age is a risk factor for later dementia, so it is important that it is treated with a combination of talking therapy and selective serotonin reuptake inhibitors (SSRIs), for example, sertraline. Many people with dementia also have depression and the two conditions can appear similar (Chapter 20), so a full assessment is essential to ensure the right treatment is offered. Depression can be related to changes in brain biochemistry or the losses associated with the condition. Unfortunately, anti-depressants tend to be ineffective for those who have depression together with dementia but effective non-medical interventions include exercise, activities and counselling.

Anti-psychotics

Delusions and hallucinations (Chapter 22) or behavioural problems such as shouting and aggression (Chapter 19) can occur in people with dementia, so anti-psychotic medications, such as quetiapine, olanzapine and risperidone, are sometimes prescribed (Figure 31.2). Anti-psychotic medications generally act as antagonists at synapses with dopamine and 5-HT (serotonin) receptors, but they can have serious side effects including increased risk of falls, strokes and early death. Therefore, they should be viewed as a last resort, and alternative approaches to helping the person with dementia should be explored first. Usually, behaviour that is difficult for others to cope with reflects an attempt to communicate an unmet need. For example, the person may be constipated, in pain, be afraid or frustrated. If essential, small doses of anti-psychotic medication should be used and side effects monitored closely.

Anti-psychotic drugs are dangerous for people with Lewy body type dementia (Chapter 7), so an alternative such as a benzodiazepine (e.g. lorazepam) would be better. Benzodiazepines act at GABA-ergic synapses in the brain.

Hypnotics

People with dementia sometimes develop disturbed sleep patterns, for example, sleeping in the day and being awake at night (Chapter 55). Medication in the form of sleeping tablets (hypnotics) such as temazepam or zopiclone should be a last resort because of side effects, which include tiredness the next day and greater likelihood of falling. In addition, these medications become ineffective after a while, so they should only be prescribed for a short period. More effective interventions include exercise during the day, access to sunlight and the outdoors and activities to occupy and engage the person. Coffee should be avoided in the evening. Light levels should be bright during the day and lowered at bedtime. Other cues that it is time to sleep include a bath at bedtime and a warm milky drink. Familiar possessions in the bedroom can be reassuring. The bedroom should be cooler at night so that the person does not get out of bed because they are feeling too hot.

Melatonin is a natural hormone that controls the sleep–wake cycle (body clock). It is available in tablet, liquid and patch form. It causes drowsiness and lowers body temperature. The medication should be taken 1 or 2 hours before bedtime.

Pain relief – analgesia

In contrast to other medications, analgesic drugs tend to be under-prescribed for people with dementia. This is probably because people do not request them but instead may communicate pain through other means, such as restlessness, which can be misinterpreted. If a person is distressed but cannot say what is wrong caregivers should observe them to see if they show facial or bodily signs (e.g. wincing or guarding), then offer analgesia (Chapter 58).

Polypharmacy

Polypharmacy means the prescription of four or more different medications, including 'over-the-counter' preparations. There is a risk the combination of side effects begin to outweigh benefits. Medications should be reviewed regularly, and the person with dementia should be monitored for side effects such as constipation.

Complementary medications

Ginkgo biloba is sometimes recommended, but there is no evidence that it is effective in reducing risk of dementia or improving symptoms. It is important to let the doctor know all the medications taken in case of interactions.

32 Anti-dementia medication

Table 32.1 Anti-dementia medications

Drug (trade name)	Form	Appearance	Dose	Effects	Side effects
Donepezil (Aricept)	Tablets	White tablet, ARICEPT on one side, 10 on other	5–10 mg daily at bedtime	Improve symptoms (memory, concentration, daily living skills, communication, alertness and confidence) for some people, and slows progression of condition. Used for people in early and middle stages, increasingly used in later stages too, sometimes in combination with Memantine	Poor appetite, nausea vomiting, diarrhoea, headaches, tiredness insomnia
Rivastigmine (Exelon)	Capsules, liquid or patch	Brown capsule, with EXELON and dose written on one end	Twice daily, 3 mg initially (divided dose), increasing to 6–12 mg total daily		
Galantamine (Reminyl)	Tablets, liquid, slow release capsules	Varies according to form and dose. 8 mg tablet pale pink, with G and 8 inscribed on one side	8 mg daily for 4 weeks, then 16 mg for 4 weeks, then 16–24 mg ongoing dose		
Memantine (Exelon)	Tablets, capsules or oral drops	Yellow orange and red capsules, with EXELON and dose written on one end	5 mg initially for 4 weeks, increasing up to 20 mg daily	Slows progression in later stages and may help behavioural disturbances	Dizziness, tiredness, constipation, raised blood pressure, headaches, balance problems

Figure 32.1 The action of cholinesterase inhibitors

Acetylcholine is synthesised by only a small number of neurons in the brain. The cholinergic hypothesis suggests that damage to the basal forebrain cholinergic system (BFCS) – which innervates the cerebral cortex, hippocampus and limbic structures – is one of the factors contributing to cognitive decline in people who have Alzheimer's disease. Other cholinergic tracts are important for attention, sensory processing and REM sleep (Chapter 52).

The neurotransmitter is formed from two precursor molecules (choline and acetyl coA) and stored in microscopic vesicles, which release their contents into the synaptic cleft by exocytosis (Chapter 7).

Cholinesterase inhibitors (AchEI) prevent enzyme-catalysed breakdown of acetylcholine, e.g. Donepezil. They improve cognition by increasing the concentration of the neurotransmitter within the synapse and lengthening the duration of its action. Initially developed for mild cognitive impairment (MCI), it is now thought that staying on the drug though the middle stages may slow memory decline.

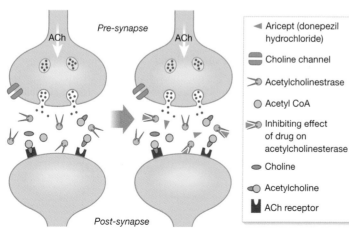

Figure 32.2 Memantine preferentially blocks NMDA receptor channels when excessively activated

Memantine is an antagonist drug that blocks flow of current through the NMDA sub-type of glutamate receptor. Its action stops the drastic increase in firing of glutamatergic neurons that is observed in damaged neurons (Chapter 4). Glutamate initiates a destructive chain to chronic exposure to calcium and further damage or death of neurons.

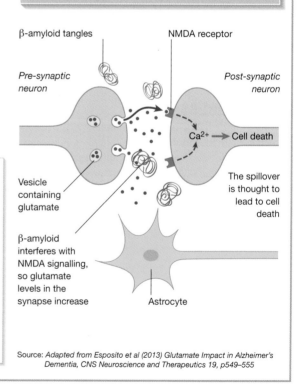

Source: *Adapted from Esposito et al (2013) Glutamate Impact in Alzheimer's Dementia, CNS Neuroscience and Therapeutics 19, p549–555*

Available medications

There are currently four medications available to treat dementia (Table 32.1). They were developed in the 1990s and were initially only approved for use (in the United Kingdom) by people in middle stages of dementia. This has now been changed so that people can have access to them throughout the condition, for as long as they work.

Three cholinesterase inhibitors (AchEIs) are available, which are usually prescribed to people in early and middle stages of dementia (Figure 32.1):

• Donepezil (Aricept)
• Galantamine (Reminyl)
• Rivastigmine (Exelon)

There is also one NMDA (*N*-methyl-D-aspartate) antagonist therapy, memantine (Ebixa). Memantine is usually prescribed to those in middle and later stages, sometimes in conjunction with a cholinesterase inhibitor.

These medications slow the progress of dementia for some people and improve quality of life by enabling people to be more engaged and active. Unfortunately, they do not work for everyone and do not slow the conditions indefinitely. The drugs were developed for Alzheimer's disease and are not so effective for those with vascular dementia. Rivastigmine, however, has been found to have a therapeutic effect in Parkinson's disease and Lewy body disease. All four medications can only be prescribed by a medical specialist.

Benefits

Cholinesterase inhibitors give most people small improvements to cognitive abilities, orientation, language, motivation, confidence and activities of daily living. Family caregivers usually report improved alertness, mood, sociability and better relationships. Even if the improvements are small, it is likely that over time the dementia would have worsened further had the person not been taking them.

Memantine can help some people see improvements in orientation, behaviour, cognition and independent self-care, which can reduce the amount of assistance needed from caregivers (Figure 32.2). The benefits usually last for 1 to 2 years, but many people continue to take them until it is clear they are no longer working. When this happens, they should be reduced slowly before discontinuation.

How they work

The neurotransmitter acetylcholine is essential for cognitive function, but the amount diminishes in proportion to the death of brain cells (see Table 32.1). Cholinesterase inhibitors restrict the activity of the enzyme acetylcholinesterase that breaks down the neurotransmitter, increasing the amount of acetylcholine available in the brain.

Memantine interferes with the action of a different neurotransmitter – glutamate – within the brain. Glutamate is both a cause and consequence of damage to brain cells, so obstructing the process of excitotoxicity (Chapter 5) protects the brain from further harm.

Side effects

If the medication is started slowly and the dosage gradually increased, side effects are less likely. They also tend to fade after a while.

The effects of cholinesterase inhibitors are primarily mediated by cholinergic neurons in the peripheral nervous system (PNS) and can cause gastrointestinal upsets, so people may experience nausea, vomiting and diarrhoea. Headaches, dizziness and insomnia have also been reported. Memantine has fewer side effects, but if experienced, may include difficulties with balance, breathing problems, dizziness, increased blood pressure, headaches, constipation, sleepiness and insomnia.

Existing medications and dementia

The process of developing new drugs is time-consuming, expensive and often unsuccessful. Therefore, attention has turned to exploring the potential of existing drugs that seem to have a positive impact on memory and functioning. Examples include anti-inflammatories, antibiotics, anti-depressants, statins, blood pressure, cancer and diabetes medications.

Vitamins and herbal remedies

Vitamin E and ginkgo biloba have both been suggested to have beneficial effects, but unfortunately there is no evidence to support their use.

New drugs in development

There is an urgent need for more effective therapies. A phase 2 trial showed that a tau aggregation inhibitor (TAI) drug 'Rember' was able to halt tangling and deposition of tau protein, with positive impact on the cognition and functioning of the people with Alzheimers type dementia involved. This drug and another 'LMTX' have now gone to phase 3 trials with a view to making them available as soon as possible. The use of antibodies as therapy offers the promise of targeting abnormal proteins.

The next generation of drugs are likely to focus on prevention, as the presence of symptoms indicates that the brain is already significantly harmed by the dementia process. Examples include medications that clear excess amyloid-β protein from the brain in middle age and that interfere in the process of its development. The possibility of medications that encourage immune cells to attack amyloid β or which inhibit its production in the future is anticipated. Research is also focusing on lifestyle factors that combine to increase risk.

Taking part in drug trials

People with dementia may wish to volunteer to take part in trials, or they be asked to do so by their medical specialist. The Mental Capacity Act (2005) (Chapter 62) guides that if a person does not have the capacity to make this decision but has previously demonstrated a public spirited approach to life, shown an interest in taking part in research, or made an advance statement indicating a wish to do so, then, if the research is designed to benefit people with the same condition as their own, it is acceptable for them to take part. Research participants (or decision-makers) should be aware that the person may be randomised into a group taking a placebo, or that the medication could have side effects. However, the person with dementia would also be contributing to the well-being of those who develop the condition in the future.

33 Medication management

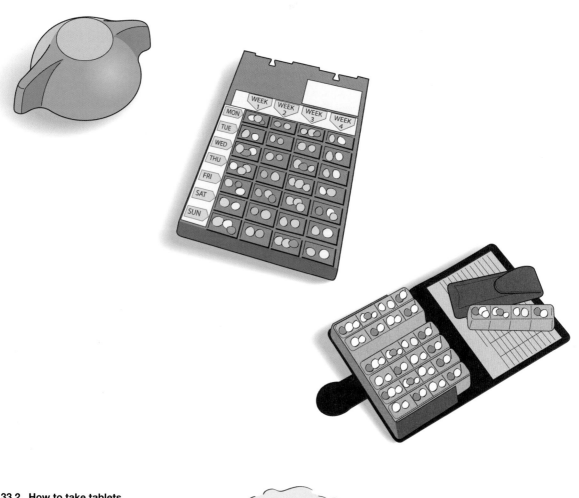

Figure 33.1   A 'winged lid' for a medicine bottle, a blister pack, and a Medi-Dose container

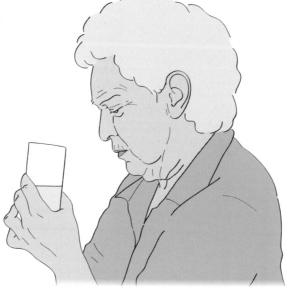

Figure 33.2   How to take tablets

Dementia Care at a Glance, First Edition. Catharine Jenkins, Laura Ginesi and Bernie Keenan. © 2016 by John Wiley & Sons, Ltd. Published 2016 by John Wiley & Sons, Ltd.
Companion website: www.ataglanceseries.com/nursing/dementiacare

Assisting a person with dementia to manage their medication successfully reduces accidents such as falls and overdoses and improves the management of long-term conditions. Thus, it has a positive impact on overall well-being and avoids unnecessary hospital admissions.

Concordance

It can be difficult for people living with dementia to manage their medication, especially if they are prescribed a complex mix of medical therapies involving tablets, capsules, syrups, inhalers, patches and creams. Failure of concordance (or lack of compliance) in taking medication can be a particular issue for people with dementia for a variety of reasons:

• Lack of understanding of the need to take medications or concerns about the medication that have not been addressed
• Denial regarding the illness or suspicious ideas about the medication
• Memory problems, resulting in forgetting to take medication, forgetting having taken medication and taking them again and taking medication in the wrong dose or at the wrong time
• Functional problems associated with reading labels or opening containers
• Swallowing difficulties
• Side effects experienced

Problems associated with multiple medications or 'polypharmacy'

As people get older and all their bodily systems age simultaneously, they will often need to take various medications for different physical problems in addition to any that may be prescribed for dementia. This makes taking the medication much more complex, and the risk of side effects and drug interactions much greater. There can also be unforeseen consequences to taking 'multiple medications', for example, taking four or more medications increases the risk of falls.

Addressing medication problems

A range of interventions can be used to assist a person with dementia to gain the maximum benefit from their medication. An open conversation about what the person takes and what it is for can give insight into the person with dementia's understanding and beliefs about their tablets. They may have legitimate concerns about side effects or the risk–benefit ratio, which can be communicated back to the prescriber. Other interventions include:

• Educating the person with dementia and their carers about the medication that has been prescribed: when to take it, how it works, what the possible side effects might be and what action to take if these occur
• Regularly reviewing medications and monitoring for side effects
• Rationalising medications, aiming to reduce the number of medications taken as much as possible and to coordinate and simplify the timing of medication

• Disposing of out-of-date and discontinued medications by taking them to the local pharmacy

Prompts and aids

Other people can remind the person with dementia that it is time to take their medicine. If no one is available, reminders that it is due to be taken can be programmed into devices such as a mobile phone and a variety of assistive technology Medi-Dose dispenser devices are available (see Chapter 44). It is useful to establish a routine that links taking medication to events in the daily schedule, such as getting up, mealtimes and bedtime.

Adjusting for disabilities

Visual problems can be addressed by the use of large font print on medication labels and on written information to accompany the medication; this information will need to be simplified as much as possible for the person with dementia.

Any dexterity issues with opening containers can be overcome by avoiding the child proof lids that can be difficult to manipulate and replacing these with specialised 'winged lids' that are easier to grasp. Blister packs or Medi-Dose containers (see Figure 33.1) also address this issue.

Swallowing difficulties

Swallowing problems (also known as dysphagia) can often be experienced by people with dementia (see Chapter 25), in which case it is important to give the person much more time to take their medications and to carefully explain that putting the chin towards the chest when swallowing as if they were looking down at their shoes (see Figure 33.2) will open up the gullet (or oesophagus) and make it much less likely that the medication will 'go down the wrong way' (be inhaled). It may be that the medication needs to be prescribed in a different form, for example, thicker liquid medications make swallowing easier and safer.

Covert medication

If the person with dementia refuses to take essential medication, carers may feel that they should give the medication surreptitiously, without the person's knowledge (covert medication). Administering medication by crushing it and hiding it in food or drink should be a last resort, partly because it undermines the person's autonomy and partly because it changes the way medications are absorbed by the body. The person's capacity to make the decision on whether to take their medicine should be assessed and then the team should follow the guidance of the Mental Capacity Act (2005) (see Chapter 62). A pharmacist will be able to advise if the individual's particular medications can be safely given this way. The multi-disciplinary team should then work collaboratively with the person with dementia and their family to decide on what action would be in the person's best interest, while also being least restrictive, then document this before proceeding to give medicines covertly if that seems to be the best option.

34 Cognitive interventions

Figure 34.1   Cognitive rehabilitation

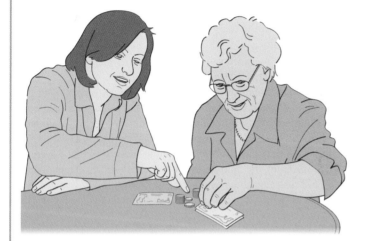

Figure 34.2   Cognitive training

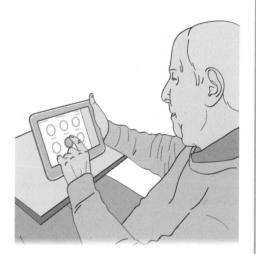

Table 34.1   Comparison between three interventions

	Cognitive stimulation	Cognitive rehabilitation	Cognitive training
Aim	To improve or maintain thinking skills and abilities necessary for everyday life. Mutual support	To assist a person to achieve goals that are relevant to their lifestyle, for example, independence within the community or managing money	To assist people to maintain cognitive skills such as problem-solving and pattern recognition, so that they can generalise these abilities into everyday life
Description	A structured group programme involving singing, reality orientation, rehearsing personal information, discussion groups, reminiscence and games. Group members are encouraged to form relationships and be supportive to each other	A one-on-one intervention where the person identifies the activities that are important to their well-being and strategies are designed to maximise the skills and abilities that underpin these activities. Strategies could involve compensating, for example, by using external memory aids or technology. The person might practice skills such as calculating change or identifying useful cues in the environment to aid orientation. Fading out prompting can be used for practical activities. Stress management helps the person adjust to the condition. Weekly sessions are usually carried out at home over a period of a couple of months	This intervention can be offered to individual or groups. The activities are focused on intellectual and thinking skills. Games and exercises can be delivered in any format but are increasingly computerised. Activities might include word-list memorising, 'peg-list' training, face-name retrieval practice, categorising words or pictures. Sessions are usually weekly, for 6–8 weeks, with practice in between
Outcomes	Groups are enjoyable and both people with dementia and family carers report benefits. However, the evidence seems to indicate that benefits are short-lived	Individuals and family carers report improved functioning and mood	There is no evidence of harm or of benefit

Brain reserve

The more people keep their brains active through a variety of enjoyable and stimulating activities (socialising, playing music, reading, doing puzzles, doing games, exercising and so on), the less likely they are to develop dementia in later life. The explanation for this is 'brain reserve' (or cognitive reserve), which involves a process of harnessing the brain's natural adaptability to create and maintain neural networks through challenging it with new skills and problems. This appears to have a protective effect if dementia-related processes later damage neural networks. Cognitive stimulation applies this concept to people with early memory problems or mild-to-moderate dementia, with a view to maintaining thinking, orientation, functioning and communication abilities (Table 34.1).

Cognitive stimulation interventions

Any activity that makes people think can be described as cognitive stimulation, but when carried out as an intervention, it involves a range of activities, usually in a small group. These activities can include singing, reality orientation, reminiscence, games, quizzes and puzzles. Facilitators aim for a failure-free, fun, relaxed atmosphere in which people with early dementia are able to meet others 'in the same boat' for mutual support. Some cognitive stimulation groups are very structured and follow a pre-designed programme, with a weekly topic (e.g. childhood, food and sports) and a format involving a group welcome, singing, discussion around the week's topic, reminiscence, a game (e.g. sorting words into categories) or quiz, summing up and good-byes. Sessions can last between 45 minutes and an hour. Some groups are held at day care centres and involve several different sessions in the course of the day. The programmes tend to be time-limited, usually taking place over a couple of months. Some have additional 'maintenance' sessions over the months following, which tend not to be less structured.

Benefits of cognitive stimulation

The constituent parts of cognitive stimulation all have some impact on the well-being of people with dementia. Therefore, when they are combined with a supportive small group, which also has a positive impact, it can be expected that outcomes will be positive. However, most studies tend to be small and often involve practitioners evaluating their own programmes. It is also difficult to tell whether the benefits are due to the supportive nature of the group or the activities, or some combination. Evaluations (Tuppen, 2012) generally conclude that cognitive stimulation has a beneficial impact on cognition and orientation and that participants enjoy the sessions, but they do not claim ongoing improvements in cognitive abilities.

People who attend cognitive stimulation groups are positive about the effect on their well-being. They enjoy the company of others, the accepting atmosphere and the activities. Family carers are also positive. They appreciate the break from caring and note that their relatives are subsequently more confident, sociable, talkative and active.

Cognitive rehabilitation

Cognitive rehabilitation interventions aim to assist individuals in maintaining or improving their abilities related to their personal goals (Figure 34.1). The intervention is therefore one to one and usually aimed at everyday functioning, for example, in handling money or orientation to a local area. The interventions usually involve a mix of strategies, for example, to include practicing shopping and calculating change, using memory aids and practising skills either using computer or pencil and paper. The aim is to help the person with dementia live with and manage their condition using the abilities and support that they already have. The intervention is usually offered over a period of a few weeks. Often, family members and the person with dementia are asked to practise the exercises in between the sessions with professionals.

Cognitive training

Cognitive training has greater focus on thinking, memory and intellectual functioning, with a view to transferability of these abilities into everyday life (Figure 34.2). The training usually involves practising skills such as spaced retrieval (remembering facts – usually personal information – over a gradually extended space of time), attention and problem-solving. It can take place in groups or individually and generally lasts a few weeks. The exercises can be done using paper and pencil, using puzzle books or using a computer or tablet. The exercises are usually graded so as to provide an appropriate level of challenge for the person.

Benefits and disadvantages of cognitive rehabilitation and training

The majority of studies evaluating these interventions are small, and it is difficult to recruit real control groups or eliminate confounding factors. For example, people who are in the early stages of dementia have often recently begun taking anti-dementia medication and this may affect their ability. As a result, it has been difficult so far to prove the efficacy of these interventions.

A systematic review (Woods et al., 2012) found that there was evidence of memory improvement in the months subsequent to cognitive stimulation and rehabilitation interventions, together with improved quality of life, raised mood and better communication skills. Participants and family carers reported improvements in everyday functioning.

35 Activities for people with dementia

Figure 35.1 People with dementia may not need to give up taking part in activities they have always loved.
Physical activity can be an enjoyable lifestyle factor that may reduce or delay progression of the symptoms of dementia

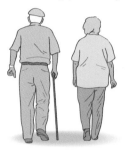 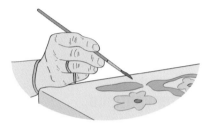

Figure 35.2 Suggestions for activities

Outdoor activities	Play	Creating	Communication
• Walking • Gardening • Raking leaves • Planting • Weeding • Washing windows • Feeding birds or ducks	• Tossing balls or bean bags • Blowing bubbles • Dancing • Dressing up • Dominoes and cards • Simple jigsaws or hangman	• Rolling pastry or dough • Making with modelling clay • Colouring books • Cupcakes • Sorting shapes or colours • Collages or picture books • Homemade lemonade • Making music	• Reading aloud • Singing • Teaching children to knit or sew • Talking about cartoon characters or great inventions • Famous sayings • Hugs • Hand massage

Box 35.1 Top tips

- Get to know the person or people involved, their likes and dislikes, former hobbies and so on
- Ensure the room or garden space is clean, warm comfortable and that the activity is not likely to be interrupted
- Be sensitive to diversity issues (e.g. diet, gender roles when cooking), but do not assume a person will not be interested in the activity because of an aspect of their identity
- Have all equipment ready beforehand and accessible to participants
- Small groups work best – up to about six people
- Introduce one activity at a time, gradually build on successes
- Create activities that build on strengths, for example remembered motor skills or responding in the moment (e.g. to music) rather than memory recall games
- Build in breaks and keep activity times within the concentration spans of participants
- Make sure everyone feels included
- Be warm and encouraging

Recommended levels of physical activity for older adults

There is a strong association between cerebral blood supply, cognitive function and fitness in older healthy adults.

All older people should minimise the amount of extended time spent being sedentary because any amount of physical activity is better than none and more tends to provide a cumulative effect. Older adults who take part in physical activity that strengthens muscles gain some physical health benefits like reduced cardiovascular risk, improved balance and coordination and reduced risk of falling (see Figure 35.1); therefore, it is recommended that this kind of activity should be undertaken on at least 2 days each week.

Daily physical activity may enhance the balance between demand and supply of nutrients and oxygen by the brain. By reducing blood pressure and arterial stiffness, protecting against damage by free radicals (oxidative stress) and systemic inflammation, exercise may help preserve neuronal and synaptic structure and this may contribute to maintaining cognitive function for longer. Some evidence suggests that aerobic exercise interventions such as brisk walking are more effective than those that involve stretching, but tai chi and yoga have also been found to be beneficial.

Staying active with dementia

Human beings are social creatures and people with dementia may retain the ability to play an active part in everyday life and derive a great deal of pleasure from doing so. Memories for some long-established skills and for movements like dancing and clapping seem to be more stable and persistent.

Activities are the everyday things that bring purpose joy and meaning to people's lives – feelings that are important for those whose days may be filled with mistakes, failure and obstacles that create stress and frustration because of diminishing capacity for knowing and understanding the world. People who are physically active seem to retain cognitive function for longer, and activity may encourage a sense of playfulness, which helps keep people in the moment (see Figure 35.2).

Which activities work best?

In general, sensorimotor skills are retained longer than cognitive skills. The person who has dementia may gain enjoyment, pleasure and even a sense of fun by taking part in something they used to love doing and which takes advantage of long-established skills and promote self-esteem. It is important for the individual to retain a sense of dignity, and this can be ensured by bearing in mind the person's likes and dislikes. We must, however, be careful not to assume that because the person may have been a wonderful carpenter or pastry cook in the days before dementia when they were well that he/she will retain the ability to enjoy that activity. Families and carers should be thoughtful about this and offer choices while at the same time trying to avoid sensory overload which may confuse or bewilder the person with dementia. For example, a person who was an artist during their working life might become distressed and frustrated by diminishing skills while painting or drawing may be a delight for another person.

Everyday activities

While the person with dementia may have lost the ability to remember what day it is or prepare a meal safely, there are still many things that can be done safely in the kitchen and living areas that will help the person to feel encouraged and involved even in the later stages of the disease. The person with dementia may respond positively if you ask for help with tasks or show him or her what to do rather than to tell. Putting a cloth into his/her hands and guiding them into the motion of wiping down worktops, cleaning windows and dusting surfaces could help establish feelings of normality and create moment-to-moment satisfaction.

It will be very helpful for the person with dementia if you simplify the instructions and break each task or activity into small achievable tasks that can be done one step at a time (Table 35.1). It might be difficult for him/her to conceptualise goals or fully understand what you are asking them to do so focus on the process not the task. Which matters more? That towels are folded "correctly" or that your loved one is dusting the same piece of furniture that is already burnished and glistening? He/she might be able do the same thing each day without being bored but feeling useful with a sense of purpose. By enabling the person to be busy and stimulated, restlessness and agitation may decrease and he/she may be better orientated to their surroundings.

Activities to avoid

Many people who have dementia find it is difficult to make choices and decisions. For this reason, complex tasks, for example, crosswords or driving, may go beyond the present level of skills; some crafts may confuse or bewilder a person who can no longer conceptualise the end product of an activity. Some tasks are quite complicated juggling acts that require different regions of the brain to cooperate; receiving sensory information (through vision and hearing), integrating and making decisions – often based on past experience and ability to predict likely outcomes – then to respond with synchronised movements.

Carers and loved ones may need to initiate activities for example by guiding someone's hand (see Figure 35.1) but can respond to smiles and laughter or other signs that demonstrate the person's feelings about the activity. Try not to rush. Allow plenty of time for each activity, and bear in mind that there will be days when nothing seems to work. Tomorrow may be completely different.

Quality of sleep

In people who have dementia, disordered sleep patterns are a common reason for care home admission because it affects cognition, the risk of falls, level of agitation, the ability for self-care and overall well-being and quality of life. Physical activity may improve quality of sleep, but other evidence suggests that exercise may counteract the progressive loss of hippocampal function that is associated with advancing age and Alzheimer's disease. There is a critical need to carry out more randomised controlled studies in the area of physical activity and dementia since a slowing of the progressive decline in cognition and improved ability to perform activities of daily life has the potential to greatly enhance quality of life for people with dementia and impact positively on the ability of caregivers to sustain their role.

36 Creativity and people with dementia

Figure 36.1   Mrs M's family model her scarves

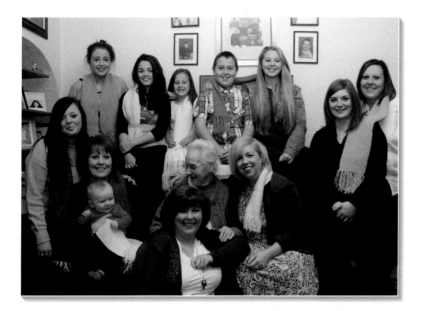

Figure 36.3   Arts and crafts in a nursing home

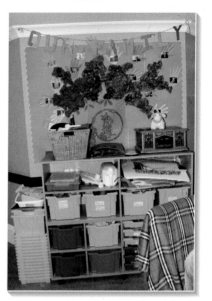

Figure 36.2   Types of memory – the speed of information processing changes with age

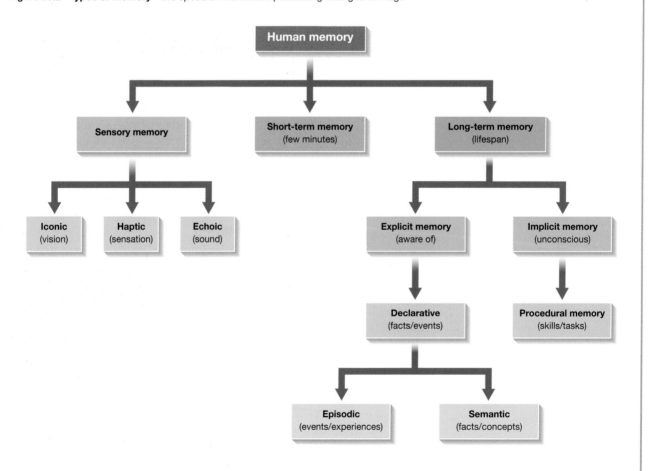

Dementia Care at a Glance, First Edition. Catharine Jenkins, Laura Ginesi and Bernie Keenan. © 2016 by John Wiley & Sons, Ltd. Published 2016 by John Wiley & Sons, Ltd.
Companion website: www.ataglanceseries.com/nursing/dementiacare

Being creative

There are many ways each of us can be creative, including craft work, writing stories poems and blogs, photography, pottery, knitting and sewing, cookery, carpentry, flower arranging, drawing and painting. Such activities have the benefit of allowing people to feel lost in the flow of carrying them out, providing a sense of achievement and engagement with others involved in the same pursuit. Afterwards, the results can give a sense of pride and contribute to self-esteem and confidence, particularly when they also provide a topic of conversation and lead to compliments from other people (Figure 36.1, Figure 36.3). Involvement in creativity can be as beneficial for people with dementia as it is for others; it does not necessarily require intellectual or cognitive skills but instead allows a person to relate emotionally and practically to the activity at hand and the people around them.

The nature of creativity

In the early stages of dementia, a person can use creative activities as a means of self-expression. Blogging, prose writing, fiction and life story writing all offer an outlet for feelings and a means of recording aspects of the past or present experiences. Many people with dementia are now publishing their work online, writing for newsletters and journals and exhibiting art works. This allows them to communicate more widely and to connect with others with similar experiences or who want to learn about living with dementia.

Creative activities also provide a means of distraction. Making something for another person takes the focus away from any anxieties of everyday life and once in the flow of making something can provide hours of pleasure. Examples might be in drawing or painting, carpentry, playing musical instruments or in work with textiles, such as upholstery, patchwork, dress-making or knitting.

People with dementia can enjoy photography and this hobby can link to other healthy and distracting activities such as walking in the countryside or going to events such as vintage car shows. Digital photography allows results to be accessible almost immediately, so the person does not need to worry about forgetting the event before seeing the photographs. Making an album to record aspects of life important to the person can be useful for planning ahead (Chapter 39). Albums featuring grandchildren, the local area, the garden through the year and so on would make excellent personalised resources to generate meaningful conversations should the dementia get worse.

In the later stages of dementia, creativity may have a slightly different flavour and provide a means of engaging with emotionally difficult issues, communicating feelings or thoughts metaphorically and relating to others when verbal language is compromised. A person who has always enjoyed making things may be able to carry on with carpentry in early stages as before, and in later stages contributing to a group project, for example, by doing some of the sanding down. 'Perseveration' – a symptom in which a person continues to do something longer than necessary – can be useful in a repetitive activity, although supporters should ensure the person is happy to continue. Expert dress-makers may not be able to understand a pattern and carry out tailoring, but they would still be able to enjoy the weight and texture of fabrics, be able to arrange them into a pleasing pattern for patchwork and take part in a group project to make a quilt.

Procedural memory and creativity

Many creative activities benefit from retained 'procedural memories'; people may forget the name of their favourite cake but are much less likely to forget how to mix one. Similarly, the saying 'you never forget how to ride a bike' highlights the way long-practiced skills are using a different type of memory, often called 'procedural' or 'implicit' (see Figure 36.2). These memories, for creative activities like knitting and sewing or things we do every day, like combing hair, are formed differently to 'declarative' or 'explicit' memories, which are made with involvement from the hippocampus. Implicit or procedural memories are formed differently, in different parts of the brain (including the cerebellum) and appear to be less vulnerable to dementia-related harm.

Emotional strengths of people with dementia

As dementia progresses, people are more inclined to live in the moment. Their memories of the past may still be strong, but it is more difficult for them to consider the future. This immediacy of experience lends itself to immersion in creative experiences. People may also be able to express difficult emotions through metaphorical expression that lends itself well to poetry and abstract painting. The writer John Killick has spent time with people in later stages of dementia and created very moving poetry, clearly pertinent to their experiences, in partnership with them. To do this, he uses only their own words and then reads the poems back to the people with dementia to ensure they feel the poem expresses their own feelings.

Childlike fun

Some creative activities are reminiscent of school or childhood play. Examples are making Easter bonnets or colouring in cards. This can be fun and very enjoyable for a group, but people supporting the activity need to be very mindful of the dignity of the people involved and ensure that people consent and are able to take part without feeling patronised, regimented or undermined as adults.

Modern technology – engaging with iPads and tablets

Modern technology is intuitive and user-friendly, so people with dementia can use equipment such as iPads for drawing, listening to music, playing music and enjoying other forms of art such as photography, film (YouTube) and dance. Music from their youth can be found online and listened to all over again, and a personal playlist can lead to great pleasure.

Appreciating art and the natural world

Enjoying other people's creative work is part of most people's lives. People with dementia similarly can continue to appreciate artwork (perhaps that of their grandchildren), music and nature. Flower arranging offers the opportunity to engage with nature and to have flowers close by. Poems learnt in childhood can be comforting. Creative activities improve the quality of life of people with dementia and allow other people to see more of their personalities and strengths.

37 Music therapy

Figure 37.1 Music therapy

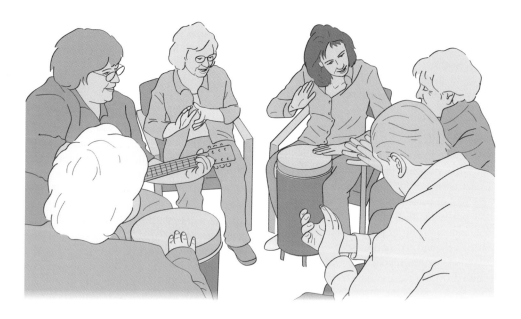

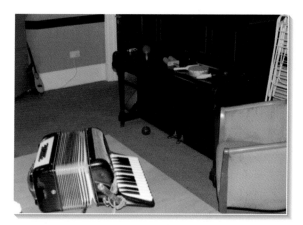

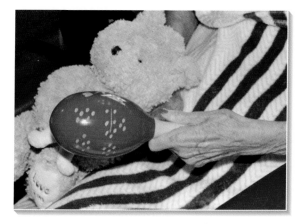

Box 37.1 Top tips

- Music is an important part of our lives in terms of self-expression, personal identity and links to memories

- Music therapy is the term used for a more formal range of interventions organised by a therapist and using evidence-based methods to achieve specific goals for the person with dementia

- Music provides pleasure to the person and maintains their self-esteem and self-identity; it can also help reduce anxiety, depression and agitation; stimulate the person and improve engagement with other people

- The person with dementia should have access to individualised music and instruments, and group activities can be provided via local groups, national bodies or social services; occupational therapy or the general practioner

Dementia Care at a Glance, First Edition. Catharine Jenkins, Laura Ginesi and Bernie Keenan. © 2016 by John Wiley & Sons, Ltd. Published 2016 by John Wiley & Sons, Ltd.
Companion website: www.ataglanceseries.com/nursing/dementiacare

Music and music therapy

Music is a very personal and important part of our lives; our musical choices and talents are part of our identity. Many people with dementia would have been musicians or performers. Different songs can be associated with various events and stages of our lives and can evoke the emotions that are associated with those experiences. It is thought that music reaches different parts of the memory (the implicit memory), so that someone with dementia may still be able to play an instrument or sing even when they can no longer speak or co-ordinate to perform everyday activities like dressing.

'Music therapy' is the term used for a more formal range of interventions organised by a therapist and using evidence-based methods to achieve specific goals for the person with dementia (Figure 37.1). These interventions can include:

- Listening to music with prompts to express emotions or thoughts
- Group singing, for example, in choirs
- Movement to music, whether sitting or as part of dance
- Group playing of instruments to tell or illustrate a theme or story
- Music as part of a themed exercise, such as looking at the culture of a different country, or a national event such as a royal wedding

Music and the brain

Neuroscientists recognise music's extraordinary ability to excite, inspire and influence people's mood. This power emerges because music is extremely good at stimulating a network of structures within the brain – from auditory centres in the mid-brain that relay information about sounds to higher-level cortical centres. A characteristic effect – sometimes described as 'thrills, chills and shivers' – involves activation of the autonomic nervous system and hypothalamus, and thus, music affects a wide range of measures including anxiety, pain, cardiovascular responses, rhythms of stress hormone (cortisol) and muscle force. Functional magnetic resonance imaging has demonstrated that music stimulates activity in the frontoparietal cortex, which directs attention and working memory, and in areas that plan movement. There may be a certain amount of overlap between the processing of multi-sensory information such as music and the way the brain deals with speech and emotional information.

Benefits

Unlike other interventions that depend on the verbal ability of the person with dementia, the ability to respond to music tends to remain even in the late stages of the condition. However, it is worth noting that underlying mechanisms are poorly understood and many studies have methodological flaws.

Chief amongst the positive benefits of music is the pleasure that it can give to somebody with dementia and the improvement that it can make to the overall quality of life. Having this form of self-expression reinforces and augments the self-esteem and identity of the person. Performing or participating in musical activity also provides a much-needed sense of success and competency to the person with dementia; it has been shown to help reduce anxiety and depression and provide distraction from pain. However, the 'wrong' music can be upsetting and lead to agitation.

Music is also a source of stimulation, which can help slow the rate of functional decline, particularly where it also incorporates exercise such as dance. Music is often used in reminiscence therapy, as it evokes previous eras and events in a way that visual images alone cannot often match, possibly because it helps to key into longer-term memory that is often affected least by dementia. Music has also been reported to reduce the agitation and episodes of aggression in people with dementia, for example, when used when performing bathing activities. Music can not only provide a distraction and refocus the attention but can make the surroundings appear more familiar. Consequently, it has been found to reduce restlessness and sleep disturbance. Using behavioural interventions such as music can reduce the need to use sedation when carers feel that they cannot cope with the person's behaviour.

Group singing or listening to music can foster a sense of belonging, and it can help with socialising and emotional engagement. For example, the 'Singing for the Brain' initiative by the Alzheimer's Society (2014b) uses singing to bring people together in a friendly and supportive social environment that serves to stimulate conversation for both people with dementia and their carers.

Incorporating music into the life of somebody with dementia

- Individualised music being played on a CD player or made available on a tape, or in prearranged content on a tablet or iPod (as appropriate depending on the level of supervision required)
- Providing a radio pre-programmed into a preferred channel
- Providing access to an instrument that the person has been known to play, and assistance/prompts to initiate playing
- Background music of the person's choice being played during activities such as bathing or eating
- Referral for music-based reminiscence therapy or music therapy, which can be accessed via the occupational therapy services or the general practitioner
- Specialist music and movement activities available via dementia cafés, local social services or national bodies such as the Alzheimer's Society.

38 Reminiscence

Figure 38.1 What may be happening for the person with dementia at each stage

Higher executive functions

Skills in finding words

Logical thinking

Balance and gait

Processing of simple directions

Less able to care for self

Declining interaction

Early stage

- Poor short-term memory
- Some disorientation in time
- Tendency to become lost in familiar places
- Irritation with own level of forgetfulness
- Depression related to loss of previous level of intellectual skills
- Misplacing objects and blaming others in belief the objects were stolen
- Some insight into changes that are happening

Suitable reminiscence activities:

- Making a life story
- Visiting a living museum

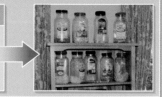

Middle stages

- Deterioratiing ability with everyday activities, e.g. reading, managing money, shopping, household tasks
- Feelings of bewilderment in unfamiliar surroundings, e.g. holidays, aircraft, hotels
- Inability to cope well with social situations, e.g. parties, theatre, cinema
- Speech becoming more difficult
- Frustration and over-reaction to situations that are perceived as threatening
- Difficulty in seeing or hearing
- Hallucinations
- Changing patterns of sexual behaviour
- Accusing those around them of stealing belongings, plotting against them, or intention to harm
- Repeated questioning due to memory loss, feelings of insecurity or need for reassurance
- Aggression

Suitable reminiscence activities:

- Looking at family photos
- Listening to familiar music
- Joining a reminiscence group and looking at items such as those (right) and talking about the past

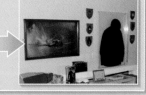

Late stages

- Total dependence on other people
- Restlessness and continual fidgeting, pacing
- Sometimes almost complete inactivity
- Person may be confined to wheelchair or bed
- Lack of awareness of the passage of time

Suitable reminiscence activities:

- Listening to music from the person's childhood
- Looking at old photos of the person's home town

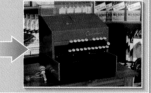

Dementia Care at a Glance, First Edition. Catharine Jenkins, Laura Ginesi and Bernie Keenan. © 2016 by John Wiley & Sons, Ltd. Published 2016 by John Wiley & Sons, Ltd.
Companion website: www.ataglanceseries.com/nursing/dementiacare

The power of the past

Reminiscence is a process of looking back over the past, remembering and re-experiencing some of the feelings associated with the events recalled. It is usually an enjoyable activity and one that most people like to take part in, particularly in small groups of people of the same age as themselves. Reminiscence helps us to put the present in the context of the past and reinforces our sense of self. It is particularly powerful for people with dementia because their memory of the past is often stronger than that for recent events. In addition, instead of being corrected about their recent memory difficulties, the person with dementia is the expert. Taking part in reminiscence activities is also very positive for family and professional carers, as they get a chance to see the person in a different light and appreciate their strengths, history and experience, so understand more about them as an individual.

Approaches to reminiscence

Reminiscence can be structured formally in individual or group work sessions or can be spontaneously carried out in response to a prompt such as an object from the past – something seen on TV or a meeting with an old friend. Regular reminiscence, whether daily or weekly, helps the carer understand more about the person's life history, attitudes and preferences and will assist with other aspects of care because of the positive impact on trust and understanding. Reminiscence can be carried out with people at all stages of dementia (Figure 38.1) (and without dementia). The most important characteristic of a person supporting reminiscence is to be an interested, good listener. Person-centred communication skills (Chapter 18), such as open questions, positive body language (open, leaning forward a little) and reflective comments will emphasise interest. Empathy also helps the person feel comfortable and safe to explore memories further.

Reminiscence resources

Personalised reminiscence resources are anything that a person feels a connection to from the past. It may be an old camera, a piece of jewellery, a kitchen implement, a photograph, a recording of a song or an item of clothing. There is no limit to what can be used although safety, space and durability should be considered. Vintage household items on a small table or shelf can be picked up and chatted about at any time. Resources can be bought that are designed specifically to aid reminiscence, usually targeted towards those in care homes. The packs include sets of photographs and may also have recreated items from the past, such as sweet wrappers, cinema tickets, recipes or seed packets. They are designed to appeal to the interests and experiences of older generations and generally have pointers to specific conversation starters for younger carers who may not realise the significance of the items. For example, photographs of Elizabeth Taylor and Richard Burton could be linked by knowledge of their on–off relationship. It is important when using these resources to make sure they are suitable for the cohort using them. Film stars, singers and famous politicians who are relevant to people over 80 years of age may not be recognised by people in their early 70s.

People in the early stages of dementia may wish to take part in building their own memory box or reminiscence resource. A memory box is a collection of personal items that bring back memories. Old photograph albums could be used as a basis of a personalised reminiscence book by scanning the photographs and then uploading them to a computer from where they could be saved on a DVD and be watched on TV, or sent for printing in a new album.

Benefits of reminiscence

Reminiscence is useful for practising communication skills, building relationships, understanding personal history (and possible reasons for current preferences or behaviour), raising self-esteem and having fun. It can distract from current worries. It can also be beneficial for others, for example, through improving job satisfaction, putting difficult current times into the context of the relationship as a whole and passing on historical information, cultural values and skills to younger generations.

Disadvantages of reminiscence

Not all memories are happy, so sometimes people become upset when reminiscing. The person with dementia may be able to say what they would prefer not to remember. That is not to say it is wrong to talk about sad memories, some people find this very therapeutic and a means of coming to terms with traumatic times. When talking about historical events, such as the war, it is inevitable that within a group some people will have suffered huge loss, which they may prefer to talk about privately. However, it can be supportive to know others in a group care and respond to others' losses.

There is a risk with some resources, particularly photographs, that they will be used as a test. 'Do you remember?' This can leave those with few relevant memories feeling left out or that they are failing, so carers should be sensitive to this and aim to make reminiscence a failure-free activity. So if the person does not remember the name of Elizabeth Taylor, it would be better to talk about her appearance or history. Topics should be chosen so as to be inclusive. Diversity of gender sexuality, class and ethnicity within a group may leave some people excluded by certain topics (e.g. pets) or feeling that their own memories are not recognised or shared by others. Sensitivity plus adjustment to resources can help overcome this.

The evidence base

Schweitzer and Bruce (2008) report that reminiscence activities are beneficial for service users and family and professional carers.

Building reminiscence into other therapeutic activities

Reminiscence can contribute to life review work and life stories. Personal reminiscence materials can be integrated into the decoration and personalisation of the physical environment, for example, through photographs, pictures and memory boxes, to aid orientation and a sense of being at home.

39 Life stories and memory boxes

Figure 39.1 Life stories

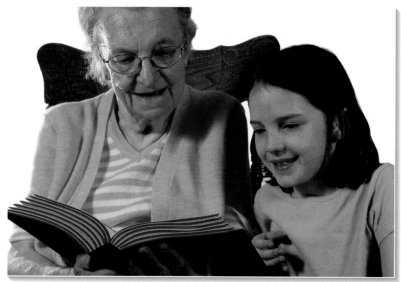

Source: © princessdlaf/iStock

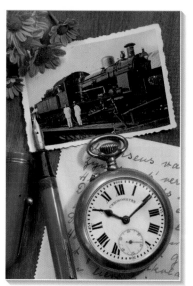

Source: © RG-vc/iStock

Figure 39.2 A completed 'This is me' template

(available from the Alzheimer's Society: http://alzheimers.org.uk/thisisme)

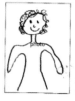

For someone with dementia, changes such as moving to an unfamiliar place or meeting new people who contribute to their care can be unsettling or distressing. **This is me** provides information about the person at the time the document is completed. It can help health and social care professionals build a better understanding of who the person really is.

This is me should be completed by the individual(s) who know the person best and, wherever possible, with the person with dementia. It should be updated as necessary. It is not a medical document.

On the back page you will find more detailed guidance notes to help you complete **This is me**, including examples of the kind of information to include. You might find it helpful to read through these notes before you begin to fill in the form.

Name I like to be called
MARY

Where I live (list your area, not your full address)
A CITY

Carer/the person who knows me best
MY PARTNER - RALPH

I would like you to know
I am right handed. I have been in hospital before but hate being there. I need my glasses to see. I have dementia and sometimes struggle to find words. I am allergic to strawberries.

My life so far (family, home, background and treasured possessions)
I have 2 sons + 2 daughters and I have lived in America (Kentucky) for 5 years before settling here. My treasured possession is my dog - Buster - who is a labrador.

Current and past interests, jobs and places I have lived
I loved to knit and paint with watercolours. I am a great cook. I worked in retail for 30 years. I played tennis and badminton every week with my friend - her name is Val.

The following routines are important to me
I like to have cocoa to drink at 10.30pm. I like a banana at breakfast time. I like to have soup, bread and cheese for lunch.

Things that may worry or upset me
I like to know where my handbag, purse and keys are. I hate to be apart from Ralph. I do not like loud noises or thunderstorms.

What makes me feel better if I am anxious or upset
I like to watch old musicals and listen to music on my iPod or Radio 2. I get quite agitated if I am upset and like to go for a walk to calm down. Please remind me to eat if I am worried.

Box 39.1 Top tip

If someone goes into hospital, it is best not to take the life story, as it may get lost. An alternative is to complete a brief version. The Alzheimer's Society provide a template, called 'This is me' (see Figure 39.2) including current preferences for routine, diet and care as this will help the staff to provide person-centred care while having an understanding of the person they are looking after

Dementia Care at a Glance, First Edition. Catharine Jenkins, Laura Ginesi and Bernie Keenan. © 2016 by John Wiley & Sons, Ltd. Published 2016 by John Wiley & Sons, Ltd.
Companion website: www.ataglanceseries.com/nursing/dementiacare

Life stories

A life story is a biographical record made by a person with dementia, usually with assistance from family members. The purpose is to support the identity of the person with dementia in their own eyes and those of others (Figure 39.1). The story may take any form; it is usually a book but can also be done on the computer or as a series of audio recordings, or a collage that is put on the wall. The story does not need to be all inclusive (which would be unmanageable) but focuses on aspects of life that are most meaningful for the person. The structure of the life story is up to the individual, but usually follows chronologically so that infancy, childhood and schooling are followed by work life, hobbies, sport, meeting a partner, perhaps having children and grandchildren, adventures, holidays, pets, the home and garden and retirement including relaxation and special events. A book is usually made up of photos with written commentary about the images, perhaps a small story of an event or summary about a person or location and their significance.

Memory boxes

A memory box is a collection of significant items that reflect a person's (or group's) life and provide prompts for reminiscing. They could include vintage household articles, postcards, photographs, souvenirs and so on. Memory boxes can complement life stories and be collections that remind people from a specific community of important shared customs, experiences or places.

Making a life story

If the person with dementia has not initiated the life story, the idea should be explained to him or her. They should then be asked for their consent and be central to its development. The person with dementia may have a preference over which form the story should take. Although the story will be meaningful for future generations, it is important to bear in mind that the main audience for life stories like this are the person with dementia that the story is about, together with other people who might be involved in supporting them.

Life review

Life review, which is a counselling therapy designed to aid someone in evaluating and coming to terms with events as part of end-of-life care is not the same as a life story. However, people compiling a life story may reflect on aspects of their life and consider positive aspects and disappointments with a supportive listener, with a therapeutic effect.

Decisions on what to include

The affected person, his/her family and friends or former colleagues could collect items such as photos, memorabilia, notes on significant events, newspaper clippings and maybe audio or video recordings. For many people, there will be too much to include, and decisions will need to be made on what is most important as a reflection on who the person is and what will be enjoyable and meaningful to be remembered later.

Potential difficulties

Not all events in life are happy ones, and the person and their family may want to think about whether inclusion of the distressing events that are part of life will be beneficial or harmful. The impact of wartime or the loss of loved ones does need to be acknowledged and reminders can provide a much needed opportunity to talk. If this later proves distressing, then the supporter of the person with dementia will be able to use discretion to focus on alternative parts of the story.

The format

Traditionally, life stories have been written in book form, as a scrapbook or photo album with written commentary. However, there is scope to expand on this by using technology to develop a computer-based resource that could be accessed via a laptop or tablet and could include audio and video clips as well as photos and script. Those making the resource could consider accessibility and ease of future use for the person with dementia in deciding what to choose, although of course more than one format could be developed. Ready-made software (e.g. MyLife) is available that aids completion of a computer-based story. Similarly 'iAuthor' for Macs could be used or online photo management companies (such as Photobox) offer album templates that can be easily adjusted for the purpose. Photographs need to be chosen, scanned and uploaded, then arranged with text so that they are easily visible in case of worsening eyesight. Dementia UK offers a straightforward template that also includes spaces for current preferences and routine.

Therapeutic benefits

Making a life story has benefits in the making and later on if the person's dementia progresses. Past memories are strongest and the person with dementia becomes the expert. The process offers structure for family conversations and shared experiences from previous times can be re-experienced together. Choosing content and designing the resource are enjoyable activities. The identity and self-esteem of the person are reinforced through recalling their achievements and experiences. Younger generations can be involved by using their technological skills to contribute, while becoming closer to their relative. In the later stages of dementia, life stories are invaluable for maintaining continuity of identity for the affected person and can be extremely useful if the person needs to change living environment, for example moving into a nursing home. The life story gives new carers a chance to recognise the person's individuality – a key benefit for professional carers. The story gives them a real sense of who the person is and enables them to see the individual rather than dementia because it offers opportunities for initiating conversations and connections, which helps build relationships. It makes care more person-centred and insight into the person's past often helps in addressing current difficulties. The resource can also provide welcome distraction from any distress or boredom.

40 Reality orientation

Figure 40.1 Examples of reality orientation

The physical environment can be adjusted to include signposting information that aids orientation to time and place

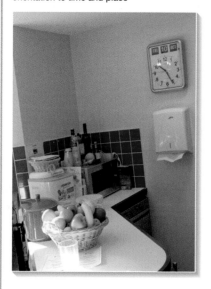

Illustrations can be used to combine orientating information with reminiscence

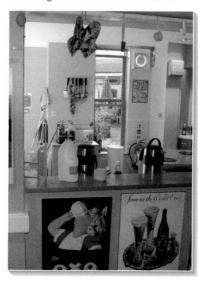

Creative décor can prompt a resident to enjoy a relaxing drink

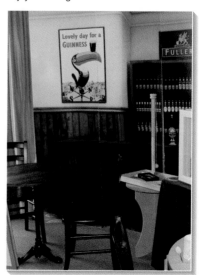

Interesting features provide wayfinding cues

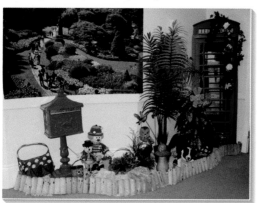

Art work or photographs can reinforce understanding of the function of a room

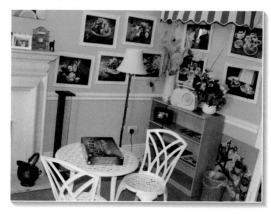

The doorway of an individual's room can be made personal attractive and welcoming

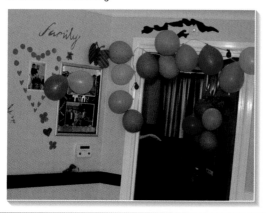

Zoned areas add interest as well as orientating information

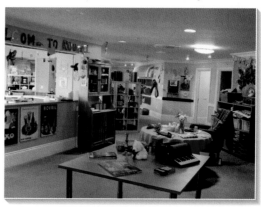

Dementia Care at a Glance, First Edition. Catharine Jenkins, Laura Ginesi and Bernie Keenan. © 2016 by John Wiley & Sons, Ltd. Published 2016 by John Wiley & Sons, Ltd.
Companion website: www.ataglanceseries.com/nursing/dementiacare

Therapies for people with dementia

Therapies for people with dementia aim to stimulate thinking, promote interaction, offer support, improve self-esteem and promote and retain life skills. The evidence base for the available therapies is still developing, as studies tend to be small. The nature of dementia means that for many interventions the impact is limited to a short time span after the intervention is completed. For this reason, many therapies are viewed as valuable for the impact they have at the time and for the social aspects that they promote.

Reality orientation

Reality orientation (RO) is one of the first interventions to be developed for people with dementia. As the name implies, it involves strategies that aid the person with dementia to remain orientated to current reality. Orientation is often referred to in relation to time, person and place. The therapy can be used throughout the different stages of dementia but is usually more appropriate in the earlier and middle stages. Whether to provide orientating information depends on the person's responses, and some people in the later stages of dementia do request and benefit from orientating information.

RO involves clarifying where the person is, who they are and who others are, where they are and what is currently happening. It can be carried out formally, in a group or individualised session, or informally, within ordinary conversations. RO boards show current information and are often used in community or hospital settings. They include information about the day, date, season, weather, location, staff on duty and relevant current events. They often include photographs so that service users can orientate themselves to who is on duty and be prompted on their names.

Twenty-four-hour RO

Twenty-four-hour RO is an approach that incorporates orientating information into every interaction. Family or professional carers take care to mention the person's name, their own name and other relevant information while they are with the person with dementia. They aim to do this naturally. The objective is to offer the person with dementia multiple opportunities to remain clear about where they are and what is happening. It also aims to reinforce the person's own name and identity and the relationship with the carer.

Examples

• Morning Joe, it's me, Sally, your carer. What a lovely spring morning it is!
• Joe? It's Sally, your nurse. It's mid-morning coffee time … do you fancy a coffee or do you prefer tea? Some children are coming into the home later to sing carols for Christmas. Do you think they'll like our Christmas tree?

Criticisms of RO

In encouraging orientation towards the present time, RO values the perception of those without dementia more highly than those with dementia. In addition, people with dementia struggle to alter their perception while it is easier for other people to come into the world of people with dementia. Some people have suggested that if every day seems the same, there is little point in drawing the person away from their memories into a world that no longer seems relevant.

However, the biggest criticism is based on a misunderstanding of how RO should work and how unskilled, insensitive people have sometimes abused it. If a person with dementia asks for their mother or a partner who has died, one response would be to inform the person of the death, as this would involve orientating them to reality. However, the person with dementia naturally becomes very distressed on hearing the news, sometimes repeatedly. RO is not intended to cause emotional distress, so the practitioner should consider the impact of confronting the person with reality and instead respond sensitively.

Confronting a person with a reality they can no longer relate to can be cruel. Carers can be guided by their relationship with the person and understanding of their needs. If the person is asking directly where they are, whether someone will visit them or what is happening, they should be answered truthfully and supportively. If it seems they are not able to relate to others' reality, then it is kinder to respond using a validating approach (see Chapter 41) in which the reality responded to is the individual's perception and emotional experience.

Themed RO

RO groups involve regular meetings with a theme, such as shopping, hobbies or current events. The group of people with dementia meet in a social way and support each other in discussing the subject while promoting each other's communication skills and building relationships. These groups have been shown to improve cognition and self-esteem, although the effect is not long-lasting.

Incorporating RO into everyday practice

RO, carried out sensitively does no harm and has a positive impact on mood and cognition. This may be partly because of the social interaction involved. It is possible to use RO in a complementary way with other therapeutic interventions such as reminiscence. RO has more recently been incorporated into cognitive stimulation therapy.

People with dementia should be offered opportunities to remain engaged with current events and reality, while also having their differing realities and experiences respected.

41 Validation

Figure 41.1   Naomi Feil

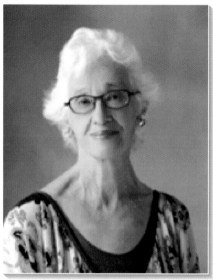

Source: *Reproduced by permission of Naomi Feil*

Figure 41.2   A YouTube film of Naomi Feil and Gladys Wilson illustrates the power of a validating approach

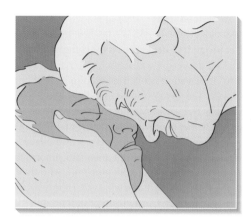

Table 41.1   Feil's (1993) stages of resolution in dementia

Stage	Behaviour	Appearance	Suitable validation techniques
Malorientation	People who are mal-orientated, according to Feil, have some memory problems but are aware of time and place. They tend to be unhappy and lonely due to anger about previous events in their lives. They blame others and do not have, or wish for, emotional insight into their behaviour	• Clear eyes • Tight muscle tone • Arms folded • Clear speech	• Centreing • Simple questions • Re-phrasing polarity ("tell me about the worst…") • Minimal touch • Warm tone • Reflect person's preferred sense, e.g. "I hear, I see"
Time confusion	People in this stage cannot tell the past from the present and tend to act as if the past is the present. They project trauma from the past onto their present situation	• Loose muscles • Slow movements • Eyes clear but unfocused • Breathing slow • Speech slow • Shuffle when walking	• Centreing • Use touch and eye contact • Reminiscing • Imaging the opposite • Using ambiguity (responding with vague terms, but in emotional tune) • Warm tone • Gentle touch
Repetitive motion	In this stage people who cannot communicate with words use rhythm and movement. They may tap or pound their hands or feet. According to Feil, they are communicating emotion and are re-living past events	• Speech unintelligible • Repeat sounds of childhood • Repetitive movements express emotions • May cry • Pace or rock • Eyes unfocused	• Centreing • Use touch and eye contact • Mirroring and match pacing • Warm tone • Music
Vegetation	In this final stage, the person is no longer communicative but has withdrawn completely into their private world	• Eyes closed • Muscles loose • Bodies slumped or immobile • May lie in foetal position • Breathing soft • Barely move	• Centreing • Mirroring • Music and sensory stimulation • Warm tone

Dementia Care at a Glance, First Edition. Catharine Jenkins, Laura Ginesi and Bernie Keenan. © 2016 by John Wiley & Sons, Ltd. Published 2016 by John Wiley & Sons, Ltd.
Companion website: www.ataglanceseries.com/nursing/dementiacare

The world of the person with dementia

Validation therapy is based on the belief that people with dementia gradually perceive the world in terms of emotional and historical experiences and find it increasingly difficult to relate to current realities. The person's perceptions may be focused around childhood or early adult experiences. In particular, their preoccupations may be related to unresolved issues from earlier times, which they need to explore and review prior to the end of life.

Naomi Feil

Naomi Feil, the originator of validation therapy, was born in Munich and brought up in an old people's home in Ohio, USA (Figure 41.1). She qualified as a social worker, specialising in the care of older people. Her theories are based on her observations and development of ideas on how people should be communicated with using respect and empathy, in order to assist them in coping with the changes brought on by dementia and in resolving previous trauma. She advocates a non-judgemental, accepting approach in which the practitioner aims to join the person with dementia in their world, to listen respectfully and accept their experience as valid. She suggests that validation has a positive impact in reducing stress, promoting communication, improving self-esteem and enabling psychological adjustment to end of life.

Stages of dementia

Feil (1993) divides the progress of dementia into four stages of resolution (Table 41.1):

- Malorientation
- Time confusion
- Repetitive motion
- Vegetation

Feil suggests that validating interventions can prevent people with unresolved or unfinished business from deterioration of their condition into 'vegetation'. She also suggests that a validating approach is healthier and more satisfying for care workers and family members.

The validation process

Before beginning validation with a person with dementia, carers or family members are advised to centre themselves, to breathe deeply and acknowledge any stress, frustration or anger they are feeling and put this to one side.

Validation is a listening technique in which the person with dementia is encouraged to express their thoughts and feelings. The carer responds with non-threatening, factual words and simple questions and does not attempt to explore the reasons behind the problem or the person's feelings. Instead, they accept them and gradually move the conversation from what has happened to reminiscence and previous coping strategies. Feil

suggests that people in the malorientation stage do not like to be touched, while those in later stages appreciate it. Validation includes gentle touch techniques that aid focus and a feeling of safety, for example, gentle circular motions on the side of a person's face or hand (Figure 41.2). Mirroring is a different technique used in the time confusion and repetitive motion stages; the carer matches the person's posture, breathing and behaviour so that they tune in to each other. A warm, caring tone of voice creates an atmosphere of trust and enables the person to express fears and anxieties. People in the time confusion stage also respond to increased eye contact. When a person uses words that do not make sense to the carer, the carer should respond in a way that conveys they share the person's concerns (tone of voice and facial expression) and then use a vague vocabulary, replacing the neologism with 'they' or 'it', to enable the person to respond again. The cumulative impact of these interventions is to enable the person to feel heard, to reduce the anxieties caused by past trauma and to retain connections with others.

Critiques of Feil's theories

The four-stage model does not necessarily fit each person, and Feil herself explains that people may move between stages in the course of a day. The names of the stages, particularly 'vegetation' have negative, derogatory associations. In addition, Feil's writings imply that validation can offer some protection against progression to the later stage. However, dementia is a degenerative condition and gradual worsening of the disorder is largely outside the control of family and professional carers. There is a risk that family members may experience unnecessary guilt if they feel their support has not been sufficient to protect their relative with dementia. Some of Feil's statements are judgmental in tone, particularly in relation to people in early stages who are described as not having completed the emotional tasks that they should have done earlier. The physical condition of people in each stage is described quite prescriptively, for example, people who are time confused have poor eyesight. The evidence base for this and other aspects of the theory is not strong.

Conclusions for current practice

Despite the drawbacks outlined above, the central principles of validation theory and validating practices are used to support people with dementia, particularly when they are distressed or disorientated. The approach offers a means of relating to the person with dementia in a person-centred way that respects their unique perspective and allows them to express emotions. The approach can be combined into everyday conversations or be used alongside other therapies such as reminiscence (Chapter 38). Validation promotes connection with people with dementia as their condition progresses, enabling those who otherwise may not be able to communicate with others to feel heard and recognised.

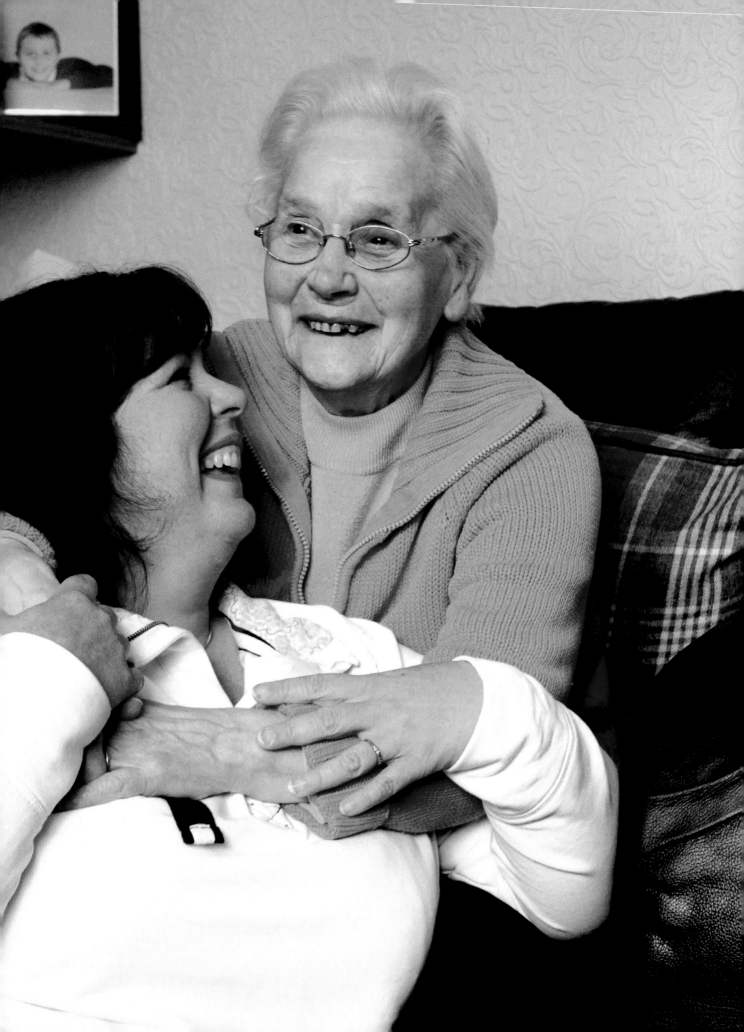

The physical environment

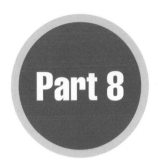

Part 8

Chapters

42 Sensory environments

Figure 42.1 Sensory environments

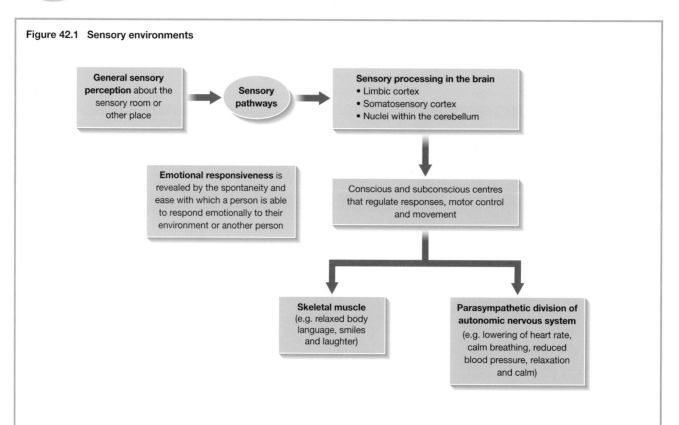

General sensory **perception** about the sensory room or other place

→ Sensory **pathways** →

Sensory processing in the brain
- Limbic cortex
- Somatosensory cortex
- Nuclei within the cerebellum

Emotional responsiveness is revealed by the spontaneity and ease with which a person is able to respond emotionally to their environment or another person

Conscious and subconscious centres that regulate responses, motor control and movement

Skeletal muscle (e.g. relaxed body language, smiles and laughter)

Parasympathetic division of autonomic nervous system (e.g. lowering of heart rate, calm breathing, reduced blood pressure, relaxation and calm)

Figure 42.2 Visits to sensory rooms, woodlands, beaches, gardens and other outdoor environments can help to lift everyone's spirits

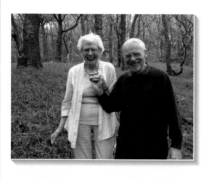
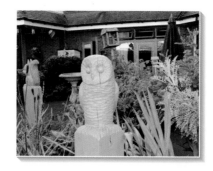
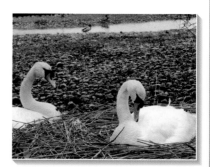
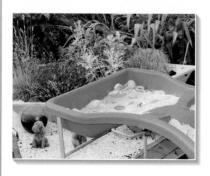
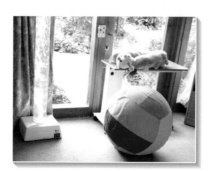
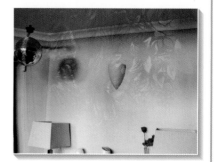

Dementia Care at a Glance, First Edition. Catharine Jenkins, Laura Ginesi and Bernie Keenan. © 2016 by John Wiley & Sons, Ltd. Published 2016 by John Wiley & Sons, Ltd.
Companion website: www.ataglanceseries.com/nursing/dementiacare

All environments

All environments are perceived through the senses and contribute to the overall quality of life of a person with dementia and those around. Therefore, it is worthwhile considering how the environment can be adjusted so as to maximise the potential positive impact, to enable stimulation, relaxation, comfort, orientation and pleasure, while maintaining safety. Hearing, sight, taste, touch and smell can all give feedback 'in the moment', allowing people in all stages of dementia to enjoy being present in a room or space while meeting emotional needs for comfort and feeling included. A room that is thoughtfully developed to consider sensory aspects can interest, soothe, support, stimulate and engage. Not everyone will experience sensory information in the same way, so it is essential for a caregiver to be alongside the person with dementia so as to ensure that the various aspects are not overwhelming or inadvertently distressing, but are instead calming or cheering.

Sensory experiences use basic capacities that are not lost in the dementia process. They do not depend on memory or cognitive skills (Figure 42.1). People with dementia often have intense emotional sensitivity and because both short-term and long-term memories are damaged, they increasingly live 'in the moment'. These characteristics mean they can enjoy and benefit from sensory stimulation. A sensory environment can be the person's own room or garden, a specific room setup for the purpose of sensory stimulation and relaxation, or a place that just 'feels right' to a person (Figure 42.2).

Benefits of a sensory room

Sensory rooms promote relaxation and reduce boredom. They may also result in improved mood, improved communication and attentiveness to surroundings. If agitation is reduced, this can contribute to reducing or eliminating the need for anti-psychotic medication. For those caring for someone with dementia, the sensory room can provide an opportunity for a shared enjoyable experience, the chance to see a person in a different way and to gain greater insight into their personality, likes and dislikes.

Design of sensory rooms

A sensory room is a room that is developed to maximise a person's exposure to gentle stimulation of their senses. The room is usually dark, with patterned moving and coloured lights projected onto the walls, sometimes reflected in a ceiling glitter-ball. Additional lighting may come from bubble tubes and fibre-optic sprays. These too can be made to change colour. The seating may be low, in large beanbags, or in comfy tilt back chairs, or a bed may be provided. Cushioning is soft and sometimes textured. The room is warm and should feel cosy and safe.

Calming sounds of soft background music or recordings from nature such as bird song or the sound of the sea aim to add to the effect. Scent with soothing properties, such as lavender, may be provided from an aromatherapy diffuser.

The various items of equipment within the room can be turned on or off according to the person's response. For some, one element is pleasurable while all of them together would be over-stimulating and confusing and could result in agitation rather than relaxation. So the nature of the room should be adjusted according to how the person with dementia responds.

Gardens

People who love their gardens will be aware that they have access to their own sensory room. The garden can be an ideal sensory room for someone with dementia. Access to the garden will also provide exercise and stimulation and if warm enough, the person will enjoy dead-heading roses, smelling flowers and the sense of being out in fresh air. For many, the sight of washing drying outside is satisfying. The opportunity to sit in a warm corner, looking out over greenery, flowers or vegetables and to see bees and smell blossoms, perhaps with a cup of tea or refreshing cordial, is a natural way for people to meet sensory needs. A visit to an open garden, the seaside or a lake, if the person is well enough and the destination not too crowded, can be a familiar and relaxing treat.

Reminiscence rooms

Reminiscence rooms offer a different type of sensory stimulation. As the name implies, they include various items that combine to re-create the feeling of a room from the past, almost as if the room has been undisturbed since a point in the older person's past. The carpet, wallpaper curtains and furniture should all be authentic recreations of common popular furnishings from the past, while other items such as a radio, biscuit tins and crockery to match the era could have been bought or donated. The effect is of walking into the past. For some people with dementia, the memories recalled generate energy for conversations in which happier times can be discussed. Items are there to be picked up and handled. These may include cushions, ornaments and pictures. Some reminiscence rooms in residential or nursing homes are permanently open for residents to enjoy as their sitting rooms. Others are more for a specific reminiscence experience.

A family outing to a living museum, where staff act roles of people from the past, and visitors are welcome to go in and out of the houses and other buildings, can provide a reminiscence experience while allowing younger family members to gain insight into the earlier lives of their grandparents. Both young and old alike benefit from the switch of roles in which an older person with dementia can take the lead and teach others.

Sensory input at home

More personal sensory experiences can be achieved in the home environment, where the person will usually have their own music and artwork around them. Additional ideas include a patchwork of soft fabrics that are enjoyable to touch or stroke, plants or flowers nearby, and tasty food that a person enjoys. Sometimes preferences change, so it is important to check with the person with dementia and adjust what is offered. If changing decorations, keeping them in similar colours and patterns will aid recognition, bearing in mind that an older person may need brighter light to see things properly.

43 Pets: animals as therapy

Figure 43.1 Communicating with an animal

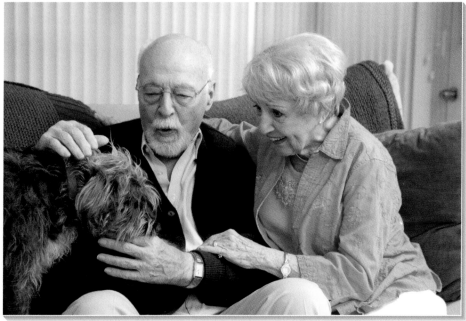

Source: © *lisafx /iStock*

Figure 43.2 PARO the robotic pet seal

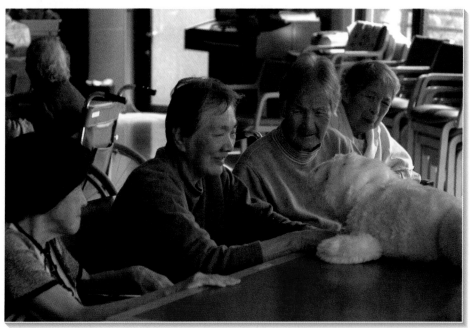

Source: *Reproduced by permission of AIST, Japan*

People with dementia often enjoy communicating verbally and non-verbally with an animal. The animal can offer non-judgemental company, a confidante, entertainment, a sense of relaxation and an opportunity for the person with dementia to be the person caring rather than the person receiving care. Animals usually enhance enjoyment of life, provide something to do or a level of engagement, and when relationships can be difficult to sustain, offer an alternative.

The benefits of animal company

Many people have happy memories of their childhood and adult family pets. So animals are often familiar and welcomed as constant companions who can reassure when dealing with the unfamiliar or unexpected. Animals would also provide reminiscence opportunities (Chapter 38) for people who have worked with them all their lives such as farmers, vets and riders. Dogs and cats are the most common pets in people's homes and in care homes, but other potential pets include rabbits, fish, reptiles and parrots or budgerigars.

The simple act of handling a pet or gazing at an aquarium can improve confidence and keep owners active. Having a pet can lower people's blood pressure, ward off depression, promote immunity and contribute to social inclusion. Caring for animals would provide occupation for people with dementia while other people's recognition of their skills would raise self-esteem.

Dogs can be trained to prompt with some activities of daily living, communicate danger (e.g. gas alert) and provide some security. Most pets enjoy some element of play, dogs 'fetch' and cats with wool or a toy. Most enjoy being groomed and cuddled and all like to be fed. Birds can imitate sounds and respond to conversations. Fish tanks with a range of tropical fish or goldfish are undemanding and relaxing.

Risks and disadvantages

The disadvantages and risks of keeping animals depend on the type of animal, the people involved and the environment. Some dogs can be snappy and over-excitable, and may run around barking, annoying people who are less keen on them and creating a trip hazard. Occasionally they can become aggressive or over-affectionate. Some breeds have an instinct to herd people. Both cats and dogs tend to ask for food frequently and need to be house-trained. If people with dementia feed dogs, they can become very over-weight, as they may forget that the pet has already been fed.

Cats may walk in front of people (as if aiming to trip them!), lie in doorways, get in fights and kill birds or mice. Rabbits will dig holes in the garden. They may also be difficult to catch and can scratch.

All pets can be expensive to house, feed and train, especially if veterinary treatment is needed. There is a risk of animal neglect if a person with dementia is not able to respond to the pet's needs and is not supported in doing so.

Some people are allergic to certain animals or birds. Care staff may object to working with animals, and some cultural groups do not accept animals inside a house or home. Some individuals see dogs as dirty, while others may have phobias of cats or dogs.

A further potential risk is that visitors (or staff in a care home) may find animals more interesting than people with dementia and become distracted from people's needs, thus undoing some of the benefits.

Pets at home

Pets often grow old with their owners, and if both are in a regular routine, the needs of a pet can assist a person with maintaining the structure of their day. Dogs in particular will remind their owners to feed them (and so eat a meal themselves), to go outside for a walk (and so exercise and chat with other dog walkers) and to make a fuss of them (so meeting the need for comfort). The pet is also a subject of conversation and connection with other people.

Sometimes older people are concerned about who would look after the pet if they should die first, so it is good to have a plan in place for this. If the person with dementia is no longer able to care for an animal and is receiving care at home themselves, it would be useful to add care of the pet into the care plan (Chapter 52) to ensure this takes place, because worries about the pet would have a negative impact on the person's well-being.

Pets in care homes

Care homes usually aim for a relaxed, homely feel, and pets can contribute to this. They provide stimulation and an opportunity for engagement. The residents should be encouraged to take part in care of the animals. The presence of animals can encourage grandchildren's visits, as they also look forward to seeing the pets.

Animals visiting hospital units

The UK charity 'Pets as Therapy' (PAT) provides visits by trained 'temperament tested' dogs and cats to people in hospital and care homes. Their owners, who are volunteers, accompany the animals. The purpose is to provide therapeutic interactions through cuddling the animals and talking to them, connecting the people who are being cared for to a normal aspect of life that they may miss.

Robotic pets

Toy animals can be comforting, but recent technological developments have resulted in very sophisticated robotic pets that are designed and programmed to look and feel like the real thing. An example is a Japanese invention, 'PARO', a soft fluffy baby seal that is able to respond to its owner's touch and voice. It reacts to its environment, learns its name, turns its head to voices, conveys enjoyment of being stroked through its body movements and shows emotions, all in the voice of a baby seal. The robotic pet can be used in environments where real animals could be too difficult to manage and has been found to reduce stress, increase engagement and improve mood.

44 Assistive technology

Figure 44.1 Medication dispenser and pendant alarm

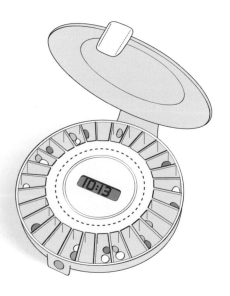

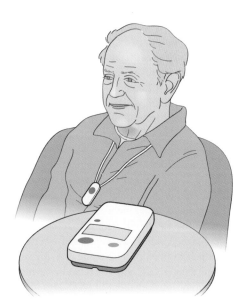

Figure 44.2 Raised toilet seat and Zimmer frame

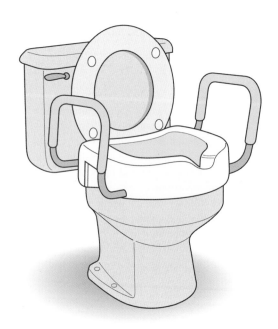

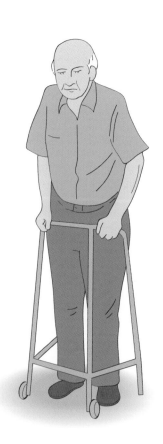

Dementia Care at a Glance, First Edition. Catharine Jenkins, Laura Ginesi and Bernie Keenan. © 2016 by John Wiley & Sons, Ltd. Published 2016 by John Wiley & Sons, Ltd.
Companion website: www.ataglanceseries.com/nursing/dementiacare

Definition

Assistive technology is a broad term for any piece of equipment that is used to help the functioning of someone with either cognitive, physical or communication problems. It covers everything from Zimmer frames to sophisticated computerised 'smart houses' (Figure 44.1). Although many devices are commercially available, they can also be accessed without charge via the occupational therapist or social care and health services. These devices have the potential to keep a person with dementia independent for longer, reduce hazards and provide reassurance to carers.

Prompting

Simple memory aids use sounds or vibrations as reminders to a person with dementia, thus reducing the impact of the disability. Mobile phones and tablet devices can be programmed to alert the person with dementia to their daily schedule and appointments. Specific memory aids include:

• Medication dispensers that alarm or vibrate as a reminder to take medication and will only allow tablets to be taken at the correct time (Figure 44.1)
• Automatic clocks and calendars
• Locator devices attached to items that are frequently mislaid

Safety

A variety of products are available that promote safety in the home. Many of these are familiar:

• Automatic light that plugs in and is activated by low light levels or movement
• Water temperature limiter
• Gas leak sensors
• Fire alarms
• Pop-up bath and sink plug to prevent flooding
• Bath water level monitor that can activate a voice reminder to the person that they have left the water running

Reassurance

Recorded messages from loved ones can be played over and over to reassure someone who is anxious and distressed and who has forgotten where they are and why they are there. Similarly, automatic reminder messages can be used that activate when a person leaves their house, for example, a door alert that activates when the front door is opened and plays a message recorded by a family member such as 'Don't go shopping yet Mum, it's still night time'.

Safety features

Zimmer frames, pulpit frames, raised toilet seats, grab rails and stair lifts can all help an older person mobilise and transfer with greater ease and safety (Figure 44.2). A low-profiling (fully lowering bed) can minimise the injuries from falling out of bed. Underfloor heating can help prevent hypothermia if an older person falls and is on the floor for a long time.

Telecare

Telecare devices involve use of sensors linked via a telephone line to a call centre. Alarm pendants (Figure 44.1) worn around the neck and falls sensors worn on the wrist can be useful in summoning assistance if a person with dementia falls. Door alarms sound if a person does not return to the house within a certain time period. The telecare centre operative contacts a nominated person (e.g., sheltered housing manager, family member) if there is a problem. Some telecare companies make a daily telephone call to each of their clients. There is a risk the person with dementia may forget to wear the personal alarm, so it is useful to encourage and prompt so that wearing it becomes a habit.

Surveillance systems

Alarms can alert carers to the person moving, for example, falls sensors, seat sensors, pressure mats by the bed that activate an alarm if the person gets up and front door sensors that activate when it is opened. However, there are negative consequences of using such devices, for example, chair alarms can restrict the person's mobility and make them more prone to pressure sores and loss of function.

Some systems include surveillance cameras, for example, the SAFE house system includes door and water detectors and cameras attached to a computer, with a telephone link to carers. Portable monitoring systems and personal trackers can be worn; they use satellite technology and ensure the person can always be found, but these devices can be removed by the person unless 'tagging' is used. Although these items can increase safety, many find these devices intrusive, and they do involve a loss of privacy and autonomy for the people using them.

Communication, stimulation and occupation

Simplified phones are available that are easier for somebody with dementia or sight problems to use. These range from those that have highly visible enlarged number buttons that are easier to see and manipulate to those with programmable speed dialling capabilities with places to insert photos of family and friends adjacent to the single button that needs to be pushed to dial that person.

Similarly, simplified remote controls are available for watching television, with fewer enlarged buttons for a limited number of functions. Some remote controls incorporate programming so that care givers can limit the channels to those that the person prefers, with a lock mechanism to prevent changes. Music players with simple controls enable a person with dementia to enjoy listening to music independently.

Interactive computer programmes can help to engage and interest the person, and there are programmes that are specifically designed for people with dementia to enjoy. Interactive computer games, such as the 'Wii', can also be used to encourage movement and exercise and are suitable even if the person has physical disabilities.

Ethical issues

Assistive technology is not intended to replace human contact. In designing a package of assistive technology, the person with dementia and those supporting them should consider how opportunities for social interaction can be maintained. Surveillance systems can be restrictive and result in a loss of autonomy and privacy; this should be weighed against the choice to remain relatively independent in a place of the person's choice.

45 Design for dementia

Figure 45.1 Ways in which design can be used to enhance wayfinding, orientation, activity and reminiscence

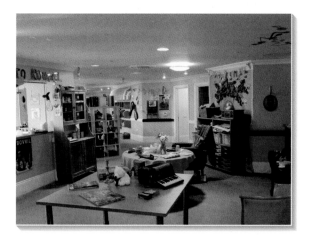

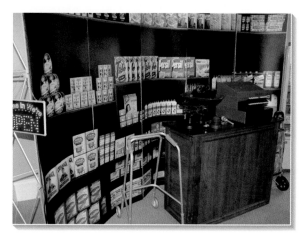

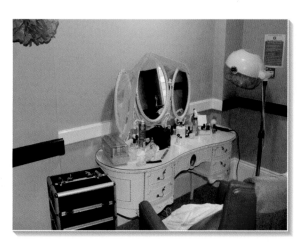

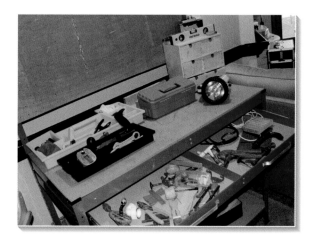

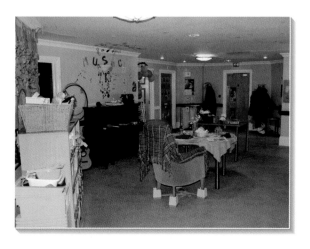

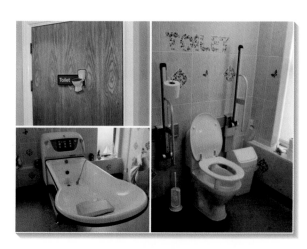

The environment and well-being

The physical or built environment complements the psycho-social environment in promoting interaction, orientation, activity, personhood, safety and independence. The nature of dementia means that people living with it are usually at their best in familiar environments. At home, the person with dementia is surrounded by belongings that reflect their history and reinforce their identity. He or she will also know the way to the toilet, kitchen, telephone, bedroom and so on. If the shops are not too far away, they may be able to go there independently and return, thus maintaining independence and taking exercise. They are probably a member of a community so family and friends can call in, which means that if assistance is needed, the person with dementia is more likely to have care arranged that fits best with their lifestyle.

For most people with dementia, these positive factors mean that home is the safest and most supportive environment. Unfortunately, this is not always so, and if the person lives alone, if a carer can no longer cope, if there are risks that are impossible to overcome, or if the person has multiple health needs that cannot be met at home, then they may have to move to an alternative environment where appropriate care can be given.

Hospitals

Hospitals are usually designed more with a view to managing acute conditions through medical care than to providing a place where relationship-orientated needs can be met. Scope for adjustment towards dementia friendliness can be limited in clinical units, but nevertheless there are principles that can be used to maximise benefits and minimise harm. The environment should aim to communicate purpose, safety and comfort. People with dementia are usually more comfortable in small groups, so an area of the unit could be set aside for people with dementia. The unit environment should be designed to give clear orientation signals. For example, each person should be able to see the toilet from their bed area and clear signs, using both words and pictures, be provided at a lower level so that older people can see them clearly. A separate room for activities, conversation, meals and to have somewhere to go for a walk improves mobility, orientation and interpersonal aspects of care.

Orientating information can be provided on a noticeboard so that patients can see the name of the hospital and ward, the date and photographs and names of the staff. The person with dementia's own preferred name should be easily visible above the bed space, and if photos or a blanket from home are allowed, the familiarity of this would enhance recognition. A bright welcoming colour and enhanced lighting makes the area attractive, as do large windows and plants. Black shiny floors should be avoided, as they can be misinterpreted as deep water and be frightening for people with dementia. Flowery carpets and colour changes can make people try to step up and over them, so they should be avoided. Doors to rooms where patients are not invited, such as the treatment room can be painted to merge with the walls, while areas that are encouraged should have differently coloured doors and welcoming signs.

Bathrooms should be designed to feel safe and warm. Traditional baths convey purpose more easily than modern showers, though the person with dementia's preference should guide as to which is used. The toilet, sink and bath should be in a different colour to the walls so that their shape can be seen. Orientating information such as typical bathroom tiles and towels can work as cues. Mirrors can upset some people with dementia, who may not recognise their own reflection and may misinterpret it as an older relative, so it is useful to have the option to cover them. Bathrooms should clarify that privacy is maintained through having safe locks and doors and curtains that close properly.

Orientation cues in care homes

If a person with dementia is living in a care home, then additional steps to promote orientation include personal signage such as a photograph or a small box that includes personal items attached to the wall outside the bedroom. Having their own furniture, photographs, ornaments and bedclothes all promote orientation and a sense of being at home. Items related to hobbies, such as knitting, or a bird feeder attached to the window contribute to preserving identity.

Throughout the care home, a variety of different-sized spaces, suitably decorated to reinforce purpose (e.g. tablecloths in the dining room, cushions in the lounge), promote orientation and interaction. Even in a homely environment, signage is important for people with dementia.

Safety

It can be hard for professionals and families to balance the need for safety with the wish to enhance independence and activity. Generally it is best to encourage people with dementia towards welcoming areas rather than to restrict their movements, as this causes frustration. Access to safe garden areas and rooms with activities helps meet the need to walk about and be actively occupied.

Possibilities for circular walks avoid confronting the person with the knowledge of being locked in. People who enjoy and need to walk can be accompanied on walks outside the home. Exercising improves mobility, mood and sleep. Same-coloured carpets throughout, no mats that might cause trips or falls, support rails in wide corridors, big windows, focal points (e.g. a reminiscence table) and pictures on the wall encourage safe walking.

Comfort, fun and family visits

Arranging furniture so that people can interact in small groups makes a living room feel homely. Pictures of the natural world are relaxing, as are flowers or plants (though they should be harmless if eaten). Decorations should reflect the tastes of the clientele as far as possible. Rooms should be warm but not too hot, and cooler at night without being cold. Familiar music can bring back memories and many people with dementia can sing even when their speech is impaired. The environment should reflect and convey positive values around the cultural and spiritual backgrounds of the people who live there. Pets, games, activities and reminiscence materials should be accessible to residents and their visitors. Welcoming spaces inside and outside for visitors, including children, will attract families and contribute to maintaining relationships with loved ones.

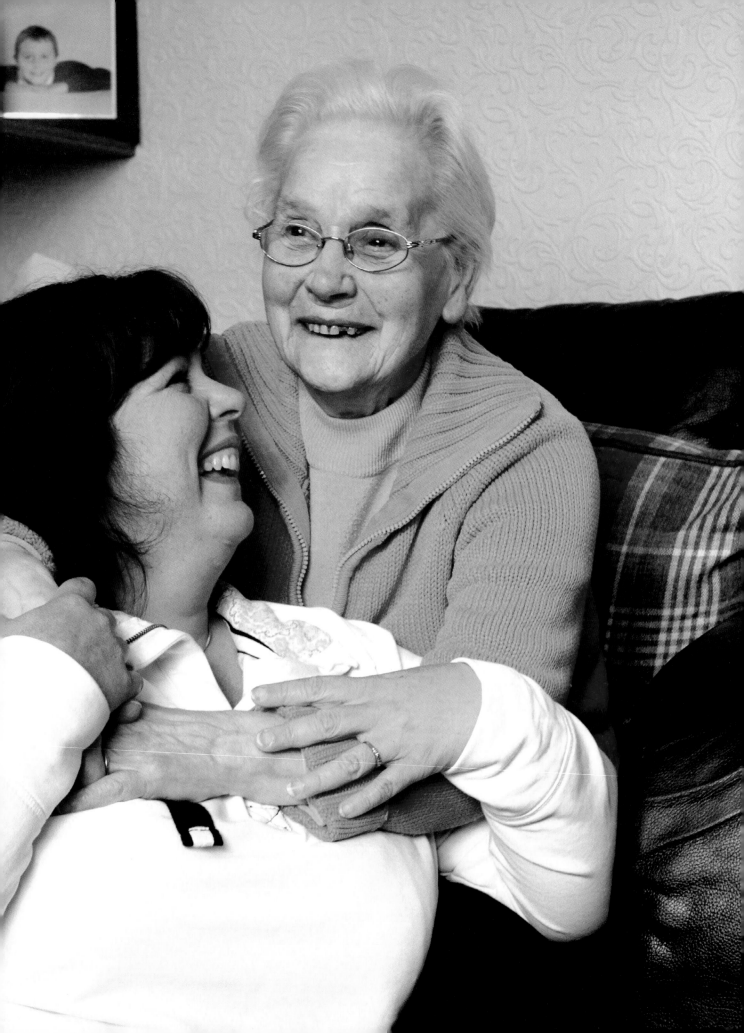

Carers and relationships

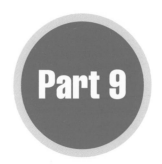

Part 9

Chapters

46 Relationships and dementia

Table 46.1 The stages of dementia

Sometimes the patterns of changes in dementia are divided into three phases or stages (chapter 38). It is important to be aware that phases and development may vary from one individual to another and from one form of dementia to another; each person is unique. Knowledge of the stages may help spouses and long-term partners to understand what is happening to their loved one, but it is often in the middle stages that the need for support becomes increasingly apparent.

Phase of the disease	What loved ones may perceive	Things that may help
Early stages	• Memory loss may be considered as a normal part of ageing • Few outwards, physical signs of change but some emotional changes • Some repetitiveness • Muddled thinking may be having an effect on the person and others around them	• Sharing feelings with each other • Speaking to health professionals together can make things less frightening • Accepting that anxiety while awaiting outcomes of assessment is normal • Joining a club, e.g. *Dementia Cafe* • Shifting of responsibilities that were previously managed by the person with dementia
Middle stages	• Growing realisation that something is wrong • Slow acceptance that the problems are not normal ageing • Anxiety and disturbed sleep about risk of accidents, e.g. stoves left on or due to wandering the person getting lost • Embarrassment about the person with dementia's behaviour • Feelings of isolation due to loss of companionship and narrowing of social circle • Need to speak clearly and break tasks up in order to promote independence • Dealing with deep hurt related to suspicion and unpleasantness from the person with dementia • Spouses and partners may be able to cope with aggression, but children and grandchildren may become distressed	• Asking for help and blaming the illness not the person • Making contact with others who are caring for people with dementia • Providing a safe and secure environment in which the loved one feels familiar • Introducing a clear routine that is easy to remember, e.g. specific place for objects, regular mealtimes or visits, clocks with clear faces • Being prepared to treat the routine(s) flexibly in response to need for change as the disease progresses • Trying to understand the reasons for outbursts or 'difficult' behaviour, e.g. agitation or wandering/constant walking • Improving levels of illumination • Diverting the attention of the person with dementia • Trying to encourage the person with dementia to get adequate physical and mental activity • Ensuring safety and minimise risks • Providing loving reassurance, e.g. hugs, touch, smiles, gentleness • Trying not to lose sight of the fact that aggression is not conscious response but may be triggered by disease process • Taking care of themselves, e.g. allowing some time to themselves
Later stages	• Feelings of relief • Difficulty in visualising an uncertain future • Guilt	• Validating concerns of the person with dementia • Accepting help from family, friends and outside agencies • Seeking the support of other carers

Dementia Care at a Glance, First Edition. Catharine Jenkins, Laura Ginesi and Bernie Keenan. © 2016 by John Wiley & Sons, Ltd. Published 2016 by John Wiley & Sons, Ltd.
Companion website: www.ataglanceseries.com/nursing/dementiacare

Promoting relationships

Families and their structures can vary enormously, but family life forms an important part of everyday existence. Relationships and feelings of trust help people to meet basic needs for love and affection, sexual intimacy, feelings of belonging and can be a great source of strength and support in good and bad times, which inevitably happen across a lifetime. Relationships provide us with a sense of self and purpose, and couplehood is undoubtedly important to our well-being. It is extremely important that all carers look after their own needs (Chapter 46). Even the strongest of couples can sometimes feel under strain as a result of changing roles.

Being the spouse or long-term partner of someone who has dementia is testing and challenging. Couples have strong emotional bonds and a shared history – often many years of shared intimacy and memories – which affect the ways in which each acts and responds when one member of the couple is diagnosed with dementia. Lesbian and gay couples experience the same emotions, but their particular histories and experiences need to be recognised. They may need clearly stated support and reassurance because, prior to the Equality Act (2010, in the United Kingdom), services were not always supportive.

If you are looking after a loved one who has dementia, you may be trying to keep going as independently as possible for as long as possible with as little change to everyday life and routine as possible. Sometimes the member of the couple who does not have dementia consciously or unconsciously makes adjustments; people outside the relationship are usually not aware of the difficulties or their extent.

Living well with dementia

In the early days of dementia, it is important to concentrate on preserving independence, so the spouse or partner who is affected feels engaged in family matters and retains their unique capabilities within the couple relationship – even though it may be difficult to know exactly what the future will bring. However, fatigue, stress and anxiety should be avoided; agitation is just as likely to arise from feelings of boredom as from overstimulation, and making decisions, e.g. related to the person with dementia's ability to drive a car can be particularly upsetting for everybody.

For some couples, a diagnosis of dementia gives strong desire to make a long-awaited trip. In the later stages, planning holidays and outings around the needs of the spouse or partner with dementia becomes increasingly important so that he/she can feel relaxed, safe and happy with travel and other arrangements. Booking outside the peak periods often means it is easier to find accommodation that suits the needs of someone with dementia, for example, ground floor, disabled shower, staff awareness. Sometimes, acceptance of limitations and the need to return home early are necessary. Dementia (and other pre-existing conditions) should be declared, or travel insurance may be invalid.

Workplaces provide people with a sense of identity, membership of teams, purpose and routine. If the person with dementia wishes to remain in work, then couples may need to work with employers with the aim of making reasonable adjustments to the workplace and recognising ability rather than disability. In other situations, the best thing to do may be to encourage employers to recognise dementia as a cause for early retirement so that pension rights are not affected.

Dealing with difficult feelings

Living bereavement

Dementia is a progressive illness and spouses and partners often struggle to accept the loss of the person who – in the later stages – they may perceive may be physically rather than emotionally present. The process may start with a slow realisation that he/she is not who they were, through gradual loss of companionship and shared activities, to difficulties with communication and the inability to recognise any familiar people.

Emotional turmoil associated with such changes in someone you love is distressing; feelings may be mixed, overwhelming and dependent on the kind of relationship that existed before the dementia. Living bereavement has been described as an ambiguous loss, so spouses and partners are likely to need support. It helps to remember that feelings remain the same; the person with dementia retains an essential selfhood that it is important to recognise and support. Some people with dementia are more difficult to care for than others.

Guilt

Arranging for a spouse, partner or relative with dementia to be looked after by others or admitted to institutional healthcare – even for short periods – is a situation that often arouses extremely strong feelings. If the admission is for a respite to allow a spouse or partner an essential opportunity to recharge their batteries, these feelings may be mingled with feelings of shame related to abandoning the person with dementia to the care of others. It can be difficult for a spouse or partner to feel comfortable with a situation that may create feelings of distress for their loved one while being looked after by others or away from the familiarity of home. In this situation, it is really important to keep in mind that the circumstances for couples and families are never the same and that we are all unique. Every marriage or long-term relationship is different.

Anger

Everyone has their own tolerance level, and spouses and partners may feel angry and frustrated at times. This is a natural reaction but it may be quite mixed and directed at:

- The general situation the couple now find themselves in
- The person with dementia
- Himself/herself because they reacted in a particular way
- Healthcare professionals who may not be able to provide a cure or solutions to problems
- Other service providers who may not be able to provide services that meet particular needs or expectations

Even if it has not happened yet, it is almost certain that spouses or partners will feel overwhelmed and frustrated with having to deal continually with things that are beyond their control. Managing stress is about distinguishing between frustration with the behaviour of the person with dementia and their feelings for him/her; awareness of this may enable the other member of a couple to cope better.

Sexual feelings

Everyone has the right to express their sexuality, but this subject is often taboo. It is discussed further in Chapter 47.

47 Sex and sexuality

Table 47.1 Problematic sexual behavior

Sexuality and relationships are usually a life-enhancing aspect of a person's identity and experience; however, problems may occur if people with dementia become disinhibited and have unmet needs

Problematic sexual behaviour	Possible causative factors	Possible unmet needs	Potential solutions (that could be care planned)
Using language that others find crude, rude or unacceptable	Frontal lobe damage, leading to lack of awareness of social norms and disinhibition. Language and social changes since the person's youth – words previously used without thought are now challenged due to discriminatory meanings	To be heard and gain attention	Take a non-judgemental approach as far as possible, explaining clearly that the word is hurtful to others. Listen to the emotional meanings behind verbal expressions and respond to them
Touching attentive staff, family members and carers bodies without permission	Sexual attraction and disinhibition. The person with dementia may act on impulse and not be able to think through the meaning or consequence of their action. Attentive staff who listen well and are physically near to the person may inadvertently give mixed messages, as closeness can be misinterpreted as sexual interest. The person with dementia may perceive themselves to be younger and act as they did at that younger age	To be close to others To be recognised as a person with a sexual identity	Aim to meet needs for physical closeness through non-sexual touch. Clarify that sexual touching is not acceptable (use the word 'okay'), while remaining respectful and non-judgemental Avoid giving mixed messages by conveying warmth and care without any hint of flirtatious behaviour Encourage loved ones to visit and ensure privacy for the person with dementia and their partner It can be useful to use a white coat when giving personal care, as this is associated with clinical roles
Touching their own body sexually or masturbating in public areas	Disorientation to place – the behaviour is not problematic when carried out in private	Boredom, need for comfort Need for orientation to private area, i.e. bedroom	Ensure the person has time in private Engage the person in alternative activities when in public spaces Use orientating information so that the purpose of each space is clear. For example, decorate the dining room like a café, have tablecloths and pictures of food
Initiating sexual relations with a person who may lack capacity Being drawn into a non-consensual sexual relationship when the person with dementia or both parties may lack capacity	Misidentifying another person as their partner Sexual attraction, sometimes mutual Unawareness of the other person's condition Rarely, opportunistically taking advantage of the person's disability in a predatory manner	Sexual fulfilment, closeness, comfort, reassurance Power over another person	Assess the capacity of both partners to make the specific decision (this may be whether to have a sexual relationship). If both have capacity and are able to consent, then the couple should be allowed privacy However, if one person does not have capacity or does not consent, it should be ensured that they are only together in public areas and that neither person is intimidated or made to feel uncomfortable Offer reassurance and redirect the person into another activity. If necessary, follow local safeguarding procedure (Chapter 59)
Undressing in public areas	The person with dementia may be too hot, uncomfortable, or not recognise an item of clothing as theirs. They may need the toilet	To be physically comfortable	Help the person use the toilet if needed. Ensure clothes are the person's own and are comfortable and recognisable. It is best to replace 'like with like'
Revealing a previously hidden sexual identity	Gay and transgender sexual identities were stigmatised in the past and discrimination was common, leading many to keep their orientation and identity secret. This becomes difficult when the frontal lobe of the brain is damaged by dementia, resulting in disinhibited behaviour	Comfort and closeness Recognition of identity and possible previous trauma	Reassurance and comfort. Maintain dignity and ensure confidentiality, as the person's previous behaviour may indicate their feelings about their 'best interests' (Chapter 62) Offer family support and opportunity to talk if needed

Dementia Care at a Glance, First Edition. Catharine Jenkins, Laura Ginesi and Bernie Keenan. © 2016 by John Wiley & Sons, Ltd. Published 2016 by John Wiley & Sons, Ltd.
Companion website: www.ataglanceseries.com/nursing/dementiacare

Expressing sexuality

Expressing sexuality is a normal part of everyday life and is an important element of a person's identity. It may be expressed through appearance, language, flirtation, showing affection through holding hands and kissing and through sexual intercourse. Depending on cultural norms, some behaviours may be public and others private. Sexual expression may vary across the lifespan and require adaptation to circumstances, for example, concerns about pregnancy, after childbirth, at the menopause and in old age.

Sexual relationships in the context of dementia

Each couple is different both before and after the diagnosis of dementia, so it is important not to make assumptions about sexual norms and needs. Stereotypes relating to sexual relationships in old age can be misleading. For example, it is inaccurate to believe that older people are not interested in sex and do not have sexual intercourse. The nature of a couple's relationship changes over time and this is also true as a person's dementia progresses. In early stages, sexual intimacy can bring reassurance and closeness, and for many couples this continues; however, sometimes one partner or both may feel less able or inclined towards a physical relationship because:

* Erectile dysfunction occurs in some men as dementia progresses.
* Strong sexual relationships are based on trust, warmth, humour, sensitivity, creativity and respect – these qualities can be hard to maintain for a person with cognitive difficulties or for a person stressed by the physical and emotional effects of caring.
* The need for closeness may be met through affection and warmth rather than through intercourse.
* As a relationship changes, the partners may come to see each other differently – a carer may not feel the relationship is as it was before, or it may become difficult to communicate sexual desires.
* The person with dementia may not remember the stages and etiquette of initiating and continuing sexual intimacy.
* It may be difficult to find privacy in a residential or nursing home.
* In the later stages of dementia, a person may not recognise their partner and may lose capacity to consent.

Sexual history

People with dementia, in common with others, may have complex sexual histories. For example, they may have had affairs, used pornography, paid for sex or been sex workers themselves. They may have an attraction towards children. They may have been celibate. Most people keep aspects of their sexual identity hidden due to concerns about privacy, legality or stigma, but for people with dementia, this may be more difficult as the potential for disinhibited behaviour can mean their desires and practices (e.g. paedophilia) become known to others. Some people with dementia and some carers may have been subject to sexual abuse or exploitation. Traumatic memories may be reawakened by the experience of being vulnerable in a sexual relationship. The situation could arise when either partner finds current sexual experiences echo earlier memories of a time when it was not possible to say 'no'. Those caring for a person with dementia and supporting partners in these circumstances should ensure the safety of vulnerable people; remain non-judgemental and calm while also aiming to protect dignity and privacy.

Sexual orientation and transgender issues

Older generations of gay, lesbian, bisexual and transgender (GLBT) people experienced a very different social climate when they were young. It was not possible for them to be open or 'out' about their sexuality or identity; gay sexual orientation was stigmatised and abuse was common. (This is still the case in some cultures and parts of the world.) Despite legislation protecting their rights (e.g. the Equality Act (2010) in the United Kingdom), GLBT people sometimes prefer not to disclose their sexual identity to health and social care professionals because:

* They may have had negative experiences in the past.
* Although they may feel comfortable with a current service provider, a less sensitive professional could be involved in future.
* They do not want to provoke uncomfortable conversations.
* Habits of a lifetime can be difficult to change, or the person with dementia may be orientated to a previous age and act accordingly.

It is important that professionals build trust and clarify commitment to providing sensitive services that meet the needs of all their clients. This will enable GLBT service-users to accept care confidently, knowing that they, their partners, community and friends will be welcomed and supported. Health and social care providers should ensure they use inclusive language and décor, model positive accepting relationships and challenge any damaging practice. The first generation of transgender people who have had gender reorientation surgery are now reaching old age. Service developers should engage with GLBT communities and plan ahead to develop acceptable responses, for example, by ensuring sensitivity to the need for private bathing facilities, support networks and staff training.

Problematic sexual behaviour

Occasionally people with dementia express sexual feelings in ways that other people find difficult to accept (Table 47.1). Unwanted sexual advances and public masturbation are often labelled 'inappropriate'. This means that the person is considered to have transgressed social norms, but the behaviour is usually not a problem for the person with dementia himself or herself. It can be helpful for spouses, family members and carers to view any behaviour as communication and aim to interpret and meet the unmet need being expressed (Chapter 19). Many people with dementia have little time or space to be private. Ensuring privacy can reduce problematic public expression of sexual frustration. Disinhibited language or behaviour should be met with polite, simply expressed discouragement, such as 'take your hand off my bottom, thank you'.

New relationships, capacity and consent

People with dementia living in care homes sometimes develop a new sexual relationship with another resident, often because they misidentify the person as their spouse or partner. If there are concerns about the capacity of either party, it is important to ensure consent is freely given and there is no risk of exploitation. If abuse is suspected the couple should be supported to meet each other's emotional needs but prevented from having a sexual relationship (e.g. by making sure they only meet in public areas). Safeguarding procedures should be initiated (Chapter 59). If both of the new couple clearly care about each other and consent to affectionate or sexual behaviour, it can be hard to anticipate the response of original partners. Some original spouses, partners and adult children may be angry while others feel happy that the person they love is content. Sometimes the original partner takes steps to meet their own needs for companionship and sexual intimacy in a new relationship as well.

48 Carers' issues and carer support

Figure 48.1 Carer information

- 670,000 people act as the main carer for someone with dementia

- Most people with dementia in the UK live in their own homes and are cared for by a family member

- Most carers are older people and have health care needs of their own

- Caring is associated with worsening of the carer's own physical and mental health

- Most carers are women. As women live longer, they are less likely to be looked after in turn

Alzheimer's Society (2012), Dementia 2012

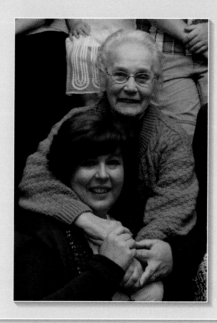

Table 48.1 Factors that promote resilience and well-being for carers

Active coping style	• Learning to face fears and accept intense emotions • Working to solve problems • Mindfulness promotes optimistic thinking and ability to relax
Physical activity	• Lifts mood by raising levels of endorphins and other neurotransmitters • Improves ability to learn from and adapt to difficult situations • Promotes adequate sleep
Positive outlook	• Ability to recognise that hardships are temporary • Sense of humour and fun help to put difficult events into perspective
Spirituality	• Help to attach a sense of meaning and purpose – a 'moral compass' • Encourages ability to find fulfilment by helping another • Fosters compassion for self and others
Strong social support networks	• Increase self-esteem and feelings of self-worth • Develops sense of trust
Cognitive flexibility	• Finding the good in the bad helps to develop confidence to cope in difficult situations • Ability to see events from a range of perspectives

Dementia Care at a Glance, First Edition. Catharine Jenkins, Laura Ginesi and Bernie Keenan. © 2016 by John Wiley & Sons, Ltd. Published 2016 by John Wiley & Sons, Ltd.
Companion website: www.ataglanceseries.com/nursing/dementiacare

arers are the ones who know the person best, and they are central to the well-being of the person with dementia. They should be valued as collaborative care partners, recognised for their essential contribution and supported so that their own well-being is maintained.

The role of 'carer'

A person living with dementia is likely to need more assistance as their condition progresses (Figure 48.1). An unpaid family member or close friend often provides this support within the person's home. Most people in the role of carer are the spouse or adult child of the person with dementia. Development into the role is often gradual, so the person may not feel himself/herself to be a carer. There is no obligation to take the role, and if there is no willing family member or friend, then care needs will need to be met by alternative people, so the family doctor should be approached for advice and referral to specialist services. It is possible to share the care between family and professional carers. Being a family carer does not mean that the original relationship has gone, but dementia has an impact on the person who has it and on those around them, so the nature of relationships does tend to change. In the early stages, the changes experienced can be puzzling and challenging for both parties. Roles may be reversed as one partner takes on jobs previously done by the other. Later, different problems may arise. Caring can be stressful, but equally the role can be rewarding. Carers need support and understanding, time off, recognition and acknowledgement that their own health and well-being are equally important. The caring role can be enriching and offer a chance for closeness and to return love and support within the relationship.

What carers do

The role of carer adjusts as the dementia progresses, and the support offered by informal carers varies according to the needs and wishes of the person they look after. People with dementia may need:

- Reassurance and explanations about what is happening
- Help with managing everyday activities
- Reminders about paying bills, keeping appointments, cooking meals and taking medication
- Assistance with washing, dressing, eating, drinking, using the toilet
- Checking that he/she is keeping themselves safe

Family members usually know the person best, and part of their role can include communicating with them using familiar and comprehensible language and promoting the perspective and wishes of their relative in interviews with professionals. Maintaining the social and family role of the person with dementia can be difficult, and it often falls to the identified carer within a family to ensure that the person is included in gatherings and continues to play a part, as far as they are able to, in the local community.

The impact on carers

Feelings

Carers may feel overwhelmed by the physical and emotional demands of the role they have taken on, with feelings of loss and grief, anger, loneliness and guilt. Many people with dementia have disturbed sleep patterns, which means carers are frequently over-tired. Carers are at higher than average risk of depression, and their own physical health can be damaged. The person with dementia may not be able to communicate as they did previously, thus leading to feelings of isolation in the carer as well as the cared-for person.

Relationships

The carer may have little time left to maintain other relationships. Even within supportive families, caring often falls to one person, which risks causing resentment and avoidance. Friends may stop calling when it becomes obvious the carer cannot respond to invitations or stay on the phone for a chat. Commitment to mutual support and understanding, regular breaks and negotiating turns within families is crucial for the good of long-term relationships. Mutuality and contributions from the person with dementia should be respected and encouraged. It is for the long-term good of the person with dementia if he or she is supported to accept help from a range of people, as this will make it more likely that the main carer will be able to continue and the care takes place in an environment where the person feels more at home.

Finances

Carers save the UK government £8 billion per year. However, they themselves are financially disadvantaged, as the caring role prevents or limits paid employment and carers' benefits are not generous. Carers may have financial commitments related to bringing up children, paying a mortgage and university fees, which create conflict between their roles. It is important that carers seek financial advice from an organisation such as the Citizen's Advice Bureau, because the situation can be complicated by factors such as any other benefit entitlements, housing and pension arrangements.

Developing carer resilience

Resilience is the capacity to prepare for, recover from and adjust to life in the face of stress, adversity, trauma or tragedy, and carers can learn skills that help them to manage their stress (see Table 48.1). Carers should be encouraged to recognise and value the importance of what they do. This includes looking after their own health and well-being through sharing the caring duties, asking for time off and accepting help when offered. It is important to communicate about the situation and their feelings with those that support them, for example, siblings, community nurses and the GP. Understanding the nature of dementia is useful, as this will help in not taking any behavioural changes personally. Developing helpful strategies, such as a diary, a comfortable routine and a problem-solving approach will make the situation more manageable and less stressful.

Support for carers

Carer support can include a listening ear, enabling the carer to let off steam, talk things through and discuss coping strategies. Information and education about the nature of dementia help make sense of the person's behaviour and can lead to better decision-making and coping strategies. Carers' views and feelings should inform professionals' care planning.

Carers should also have a clear idea of where to get help and what help is available. Respite care, day care, sitting services, carers groups and local voluntary services can all be helpful. Carers are entitled to a separate assessment of their own needs. This includes finances and information about how to access a package of support.

49 Reducing stress levels for family carers

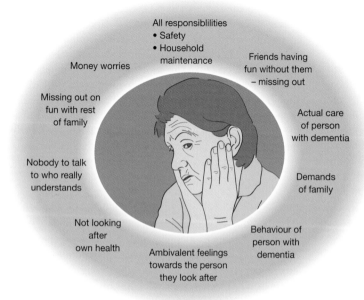

Figure 49.1 Family carer stressors

- All responsiblilities
  - Safety
  - Household maintenance
- Friends having fun without them – missing out
- Money worries
- Missing out on fun with rest of family
- Actual care of person with dementia
- Nobody to talk to who really understands
- Demands of family
- Not looking after own health
- Behaviour of person with dementia
- Ambivalent feelings towards the person they look after

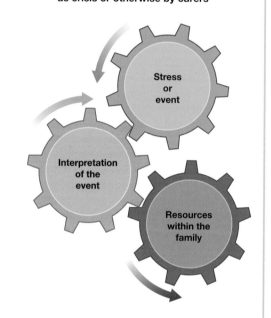

Figure 49.2 A dynamic interplay between factors will determine whether an event is perceived as crisis or otherwise by carers

- Stress or event
- Interpretation of the event
- Resources within the family

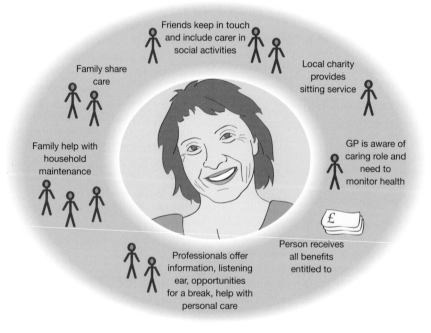

Figure 49.3 Supporting factors/network

- Friends keep in touch and include carer in social activities
- Family share care
- Local charity provides sitting service
- Family help with household maintenance
- GP is aware of caring role and need to monitor health
- Professionals offer information, listening ear, opportunities for a break, help with personal care
- Person receives all benefits entitled to

If someone moves into a care home…

- Family carers may not feel the relief expected
- Aim to relate well to care home staff. Collaborate, support when monitoring, offer positive feedback, help them see the history and preferences of the person, so it is easier for them to recognise them as a person, show appreciation

For paid carers in a care home…

- If you are working in a home, show appreciation, ensure regular proper breaks, support colleagues, aim to take an empathic problem-solving approach, acknowledge the multiple roles you play: guide, interpreter, parent, detective, entertainer, health and safety monitor, waiter, butler, sensitive provider of personal care – don't underestimate your skills and consider own well-being

Dementia Care at a Glance, First Edition. Catharine Jenkins, Laura Ginesi and Bernie Keenan. © 2016 by John Wiley & Sons, Ltd. Published 2016 by John Wiley & Sons, Ltd.
Companion website: www.ataglanceseries.com/nursing/dementiacare

Stressors

Family carers may find they are involved in making more decisions, coping with roles previously taken by a partner (such as paying bills, doing housework) and facing problems previously dealt with as a couple or alone (Figure 49.1). If the person's condition worsens, family carers could find themselves taking on additional responsibilities:

- For safety (e.g. checking if the gas is off)
- Planning ahead for simple (e.g. what to have for dinner) and more complicated issues (e.g. how to maintain the home)
- Managing relationships with others outside the family

The role of a carer may gradually involve more practical assistance, for example:

- Washing and dressing the person with dementia
- Making sure he/she drinks and eats enough
- Ensuring that he/she manages using the toilet

Mutual understanding can become difficult when the person with dementia is less able to express their needs and to understand what other people are saying. Sometimes people with dementia communicate distress through behaviour that is difficult for others to cope with, or they may become uncharacteristically disinhibited or apathetic. Emotional issues such as anxious and agitated behaviour (crying, following and repetitive questioning) (see Chapter 19) can be harder for carers than the physical demands of caring such as assistance with bathing.

- Caring for a relative can strain marital relationships, as the spouse may feel neglected or that the carer is prioritising a parent over children.
- If a family member has to give up work in order to care, this can cause financial difficulties and debt.
- Isolated carers may worry about what might happen to their loved one if they themselves were to become ill or die.

Sharing care

Family structures differ and care may be shared within a family or fall mainly on one person's shoulders. In nuclear families, a spouse, partner or adult child may be the main carer with the support of other members, while in an extended family care may be shared more equally between relatives. Family belief systems and interconnectedness are important when discussing problem-solving plans for future care (Figure 49.2). Some families have a more collaborative organisational structure than others.

Honest conversations about the future

When considering how dementia may progress, it is important for all parties to be mutually supportive and honest about how much they will be able to contribute. As care may become stressful, it is vital that families consider as a group how they will support a main carer and liaise with service providers from health and social care sector.

The person with dementia is central to discussions and should be asked how they feel about alternative plans. Caring may last many years, so the welfare of carers is as important of that of the person they look after. Overwhelming stress can lead to ill-health in the carer and the decision to give up caring, while shared, mutually supportive caring arrangements are more likely to result in the person with dementia and their family continuing in an arrangement that they choose.

Coping strategies

Family carers need the support of those closest to them; thus, they should be encouraged to accept support from other family members, friends and from within their communities, for example, faith organisations (Figure 49.3).

Support from services

A variety of support services may be available in the local area. These can include admiral nurses (specialist nurses whose role is to support family carers); community mental health teams; day care, respite and sitting services; carer support groups; Alzheimer's cafes and voluntary organisations' input. Carers have the right to an assessment of their own needs from their local authority. This means a social worker would have a structured conversation about the situation and what benefits and assistance could be provided.

Self-support and mutual support

Some caregivers are more resilient and able to cope with the challenge of looking after a loved one with dementia than others. Resilience is about an individual's protection from stress and ability to grow and develop from difficult circumstances (bounce forward). Factors that promote resilience include being optimistic, having a sense of moral compass or purpose, feelings of courage, physical and mental fitness and flexibility. A strong social support network is important. Feeling resilient and positive makes the job easier, so carers should take all opportunities available to maintain and improve their own health and well-being.

Both the main carer and their support network should recognise how important it is to:

- Take a break: This helps the carer relax and enables the person with dementia to accept help from others.
- Eat healthily and take exercise: Caring is physically and emotionally tiring; a stronger and well-nourished carer is better able to cope.
- Be kind to themselves: Think how they might advise a good friend in the same situation and act accordingly.
- Get good information: Understanding the condition and the reasons for changes helps a carer not to take things personally. The Alzheimer's Society is a useful source.
- Maintain relationships and connections to their community.
- Accept comfort support and any contributions from the cared-for person, aim for a mutually caring relationship.
- Accept offers of help: Doing this often means that others carry on offering later when it might be needed more.
- Consider what the person cared-for might say about the carer's needs.
- Reflect on the meaningfulness of the role, for example, in keeping a promise or accepting a religious duty. Caring can be spiritually culturally and personally satisfying.

50 Having difficult conversations

Table 50.1 Strategies for coping with emotionally upsetting conversations

Statement/conversation topic	Possible feelings or reasons	Suggested responses
Calling for mother	• Fear • Abandonment • Need for reassurance	• Reassurance that although the person they are calling for is not around, there is still someone caring nearby who will make sure they are safe
At certain times of day, wanting to go to the school to collect young children or to go home to put their partner's dinner on	• Triggered by routine, a sense of responsibility, a need to be needed or have a role • Boredom • Restless legs syndrome or a need for exercise/walking • A sense that there is something wrong and a feeling that an old role will contribute to making things feel right again	• If the person seems to need to be occupied, they can be involved in a useful activity and thanked for their part in this • More opportunities for exercise and walking • Reassurance and explanation of the day's activities • Visual cues to location and purpose within the built environment
Wanting to return to their own childhood home	• Not recognising current surroundings (particularly late afternoon when light levels go and they feel tired). Looking for somewhere recognisable and safe	• Acknowledging strangeness, e.g. 'Even though you've lived here a while, it still seems strange sometimes?' • Walking outside more in the day time, returning to current home and a welcome plus hot drink • 'Tell me more about where you used to live…' plus validation, e.g. 'Sounds like you miss it..'
Asking to die, or "When will the Lord take me"	• Being in pain • Possible low mood (Chapter 20) • Missing departed friends and family • Genuine enquiry	• Treat pain with analgesia • Ask about mood – 'sounds like you're feeling fed up… is there anything I can do?' • Respond with warmth and concern, e.g. 'Are you feeling he's overlooked you?' • Reassurance about being valued and cared for. Aim to respond congruently with the person's belief system. Ask if they would like to speak with a chaplain as well. Aim to spend more time with them even though the conversations may be difficult • Answer health-related questions simply and honestly, e.g. 'You're right, you are very poorly, but I don't know when you will go'. Comfort
Misrecognition, e.g. their own reflection or photograph as their parent or grandparent, or son as father	• Unawareness of their current appearance (feeling younger or as a child). Seeing a family likeness. Feelings could be mixed – joy, shock, etc.	• Respond to feeling: was it a bit of a shock to see an old lady looking like …? Plus reassurance – 'Don't worry, it was the mirror' (plan to cover or remove mirror) • 'Your son must look like your own Dad – are they alike in character?' Reassurance and comfort

Dementia Care at a Glance, First Edition. Catharine Jenkins, Laura Ginesi and Bernie Keenan. © 2016 by John Wiley & Sons, Ltd. Published 2016 by John Wiley & Sons, Ltd.
Companion website: www.ataglanceseries.com/nursing/dementiacare

Introduction

One of the benefits of earlier diagnosis of dementia is the chance to have conversations about things that matter now and are anticipated to matter in the future. Looking forward to a time when one may not have capacity to make decisions, to recognise loved ones or to respond 'in character' can be difficult for the person who has been given a diagnosis of dementia and for those supporting them. Planning ahead together for the future should result in greater peace of mind due to mutual understanding of priorities and improved clarity about future decision-making. Professionals build expertise in coping with difficult conversations, whereas family members are unlikely to have this experience. Perception of difficulty varies, so what is perceived as difficult for one may be less challenging for another.

Planning ahead

Honest conversations about the future are the basis of clear decision-making later. The person with dementia should be involved in conversations about the future, unless they decline. Things that need to be discussed may be difficult as they acknowledge current stress and the difficulties of what may lie ahead, but addressing potentially sensitive issues and clearing the air should bring reassurance and lead to closer, more supportive and understanding relationships.

Topics to be considered are the person's wishes for the next stages of their life and after their death. If a will has not been made, then this should be considered a priority while the person is able to express their wishes and understand the consequences of decisions (that is while they have capacity for this). Similarly 'living will' or 'advance decisions' should be made while the person is able to consider what they would prefer should their health deteriorate to the point where they will need assistance with daily activities and decision-making. The person with dementia could consider where they would prefer to live, who they would like to be involved in their care and what treatment they would accept and refuse. Sometimes people choose, in an 'advance directive' to refuse life-saving treatments, for example, artificial feeding, life support (see Chapter 62).

It is possible to live well with dementia, and the person recently diagnosed should be reassured about family relationships and that, if needed, good-quality professional care will be found. However, the person may wish to discuss assisted suicide or euthanasia (neither of which are legal in the United Kingdom) – listening and reassuring about future support may put their mind at rest. It is a good idea to identify trusted people who could be involved in decision-making, should the person become unable to do this independently (see Chapter 62). Planning should take into account whether potential supporters are willing and able to take on roles as decision-makers, for example, through a 'lasting power of attorney'.

Emotional distress

Different types of difficult conversations tend to arise as the condition progresses. If the person feels unsafe, lonely, bored or without a role, then statements may reflect feelings to which others can respond. Examples are given in Table 50.1.

Truth-telling or 'therapeutic lies'

Repeatedly breaking bad news can lead to recurring grief or a sense of humiliation when misunderstandings are clarified. Professional and family caregivers often come to the conclusion that there is no point in confronting the person with reality when it is so distressing. To avoid this, sometimes 'white lies' are used to distract or mislead, such as 'He's at work', 'The neighbour is collecting them today' or 'You're staying with us for a while'. Although each person is different, there is a risk of breaking trust or creating frustration. Generally it is better to acknowledge and validate feelings, for example, 'You really love him don't you?' followed by emotional support.

Reliving trauma

Sometimes speech and behaviour show that a person is reliving traumatic memories from their youth. For example, those who lived through the war can become very distressed by fear of aerial bombing and insist that lights are turned off when it is dark. Sometimes their behaviour when assisted with washing indicates possible childhood sexual abuse. Compassionate responses include making changes to routines such as closing curtains, different gender of caregiver together with cues that demonstrate a secure reality (e.g. nurses' uniform) together with a calm reassuring approach.

Mistaken identity

Family likenesses can lead to upsetting instances of misrecognition. If a person feels as if they are a child themselves, then it is logical that their son may be misrecognised as a sibling or even father. Though upsetting, a more positive view could be that even in a state of confusion, the person is able to recognise a family relationship.

Disinhibition

Damage to the frontal lobe can lead to disinhibition and uncharacteristic use of language. Swearing is an example, and while relatives may be shocked, this behaviour is not evidence of a personality change, it is more an indication of direct expression of feelings. It is best to avoid judgement or 'telling the person off' and respond to their feelings.

Word-finding difficulties and frustration

When someone cannot find the right word or is unable to make himself or herself understood, it can be extremely frustrating. Most people with dementia with word-finding difficulties say they would rather try by themselves, then be offered alternatives if unsuccessful. Acknowledging frustration and then suggesting 'You can come back to it later, if you want to' can help.

Lack of conversation – mutism

It can be difficult to keep talking when there is no response, as sometimes happens when people are during the later stages of dementia. Mutism can lead other people to avoid the company of the person with dementia, which leads to isolation. However, lack of verbal response does not equal lack of feeling, and it is best to include the person through non-verbal communication, demonstrating warmth through facial expressions, tone of voice and holding their hand.

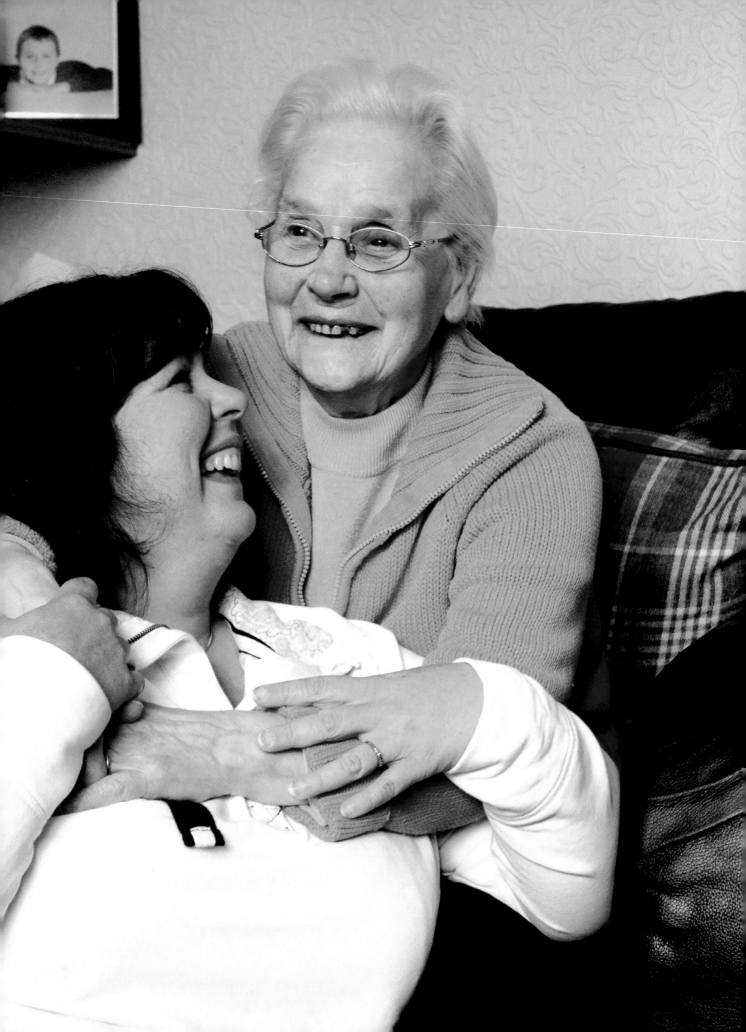

Responding to dementia-related difficulties

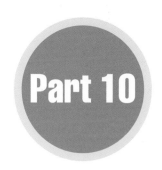
Part 10

Chapters

51 The multi-disciplinary team

Figure 51.1 Dementia pathway

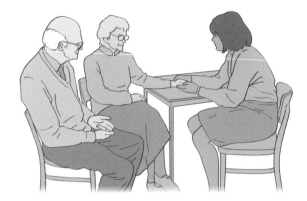

GP family practice

- Specialist nurse
- Consultant psychiatrist
- CT scanning
- Memory clinic

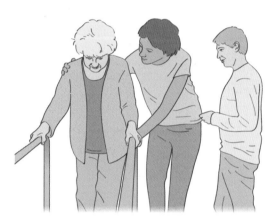

At home

- Community mental health nurse
- Voluntary organisation worker (at home or in social settings)
- Admiral Nurse (for carer support)
- Occupational therapist (OT)
- Physiotherapist
- Social worker
- Home carer
- Speech and language therapist (SALT)

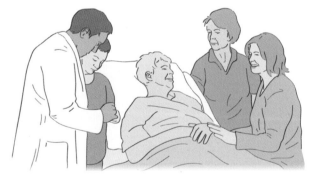

In hospital/care home

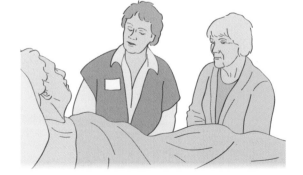

Hospice

Dementia Care at a Glance, First Edition. Catharine Jenkins, Laura Ginesi and Bernie Keenan. © 2016 by John Wiley & Sons, Ltd. Published 2016 by John Wiley & Sons, Ltd.
Companion website: www.ataglanceseries.com/nursing/dementiacare

Before meeting the multi-disciplinary team

The person who has been experiencing difficulties with their memory, concentration or mood (and their family members) may have been feeling anxious about these issues for some time before they meet any health and social care professionals. Timely sensitive support and guidance throughout the assessment, treatment and care that is offered by the team will enable them to gain maximum benefit (Figure 51.1). The person with dementia, together with supportive others who they trust, should be involved in every stage and decision. Before making contact, the family will probably have researched some issues online and may have weighed up advantages and disadvantages of gaining a diagnosis. They may also feel scared of what could lie ahead. Honest but sensitive responses, expressed in normal language, are required. The person who may have dementia also has the right to decide not to seek a diagnosis and not to take the support offered. However, the benefits of an early diagnosis and accepting help when needed do make living with dementia easier for the one who has the condition and those who are close to them. This is more effective when they are both included as partners in care planning and delivery.

First point of contact

The first person to contact about concerns is the family doctor, or general practitioner (GP), who may appreciate a longer appointment time to carry out the assessment. The GP will 'take a history' or find out what has been happening and for how long. They will probably also take blood samples to help them rule out any treatable conditions that can mimic dementia (such as thyroid problems). They may ask a series of questions about memory and mood, and ask the person to take part in a brief assessment such as the '6CIT' or MMSE (Chapter 11). If the GP concludes that the memory problems could be related to dementia, they will then probably ask their patient's permission to make a referral to a memory clinic. They may also be able to 'signpost' to local sources of information and support (Chapter 13).

Unfortunately, not all GPs are confident in diagnosing dementia, and occasionally they may believe that a diagnosis is not helpful (due to the anxiety and stigma that can be involved) or the false belief that there is no useful treatment. A diagnosis enables access to other services and benefits, together with an opportunity for the person and their family to discuss decisions about the future.

The memory clinic

Memory clinics are led by consultant psychiatrists who specialise in the assessment and treatment of people with dementia. The multi-disciplinary assessment process will involve the person with dementia (and the person supporting them, who is encouraged to come with them) meeting the following professionals:

• A friendly, dementia-sensitive receptionist
• A mental health nurse, who may explain what to expect and offer pre-diagnostic counselling
• A doctor, either the consultant or a member of the medical team, who will take a detailed history, assess more thoroughly and may prescribe anti-dementia medication

• Relevant professionals who may be involved to take blood samples (phlebotomist) carry out a brain scan (diagnostic radiologist) and electrocardiogram (nurse or doctor)

Memory clinic patients may also see or be referred to:

• A psychologist or nurse, who can explain more about the condition, suggest coping strategies and may offer a cognitive stimulation group. They may discuss planning ahead and concerns about driving and legal issues
• An occupational therapist, who can advise on maintaining independence, assistive technology and home adjustments
• A social worker, who can explain options for on-going care, if needed
• A representative of a local voluntary group who can offer contact details and information about other support

Following assessment, the multi-disciplinary team will arrange follow-up appointments.

Support at home

Most people with dementia live at home, either independently or with some degree of support from family friends and professionals. A **community mental health nurse's** (CMHN) role is to carry out assessments, advise on medication, discuss problems, offer advice and support and liaise with others in the team to ensure they work together smoothly. **Admiral nurses** are not available in all areas; their specialist role is to support carers. They offer counselling, signposting and advice. If the person with dementia needs assistance with personal care, a **social worker** would carry out an assessment of needs, assist in designing a package of care and advise on personal budgets and direct payments. **Home carers** could be involved in helping with washing, dressing, meeting dietary and toileting needs. Respite care could be offered. If there are concerns that the person with dementia is at risk, the social worker would take the lead in a safeguarding response (Chapter 59). This may include offering more support to reduce any contributing stress.

Nursing home care, hospital or hospice

If care needs increase, these professionals could offer advice:

• Nurses and health care assistants to provide care
• A nutritionist: on diet and nutrition
• A speech and language therapist (SALT): on communication and swallowing difficulties
• Psychiatric liaison teams in general hospitals
• An activity worker: on therapeutic activities
• A physiotherapist on movement and mobility
• A chaplain: on spiritual concerns
• A pharmacist: on medication prescription and management
• Palliative care and pain management specialists: on end-of-life care

The multi-disciplinary team aim to work together with people affected by dementia and their families offering advice, support care and treatment throughout the condition.

52 Care planning

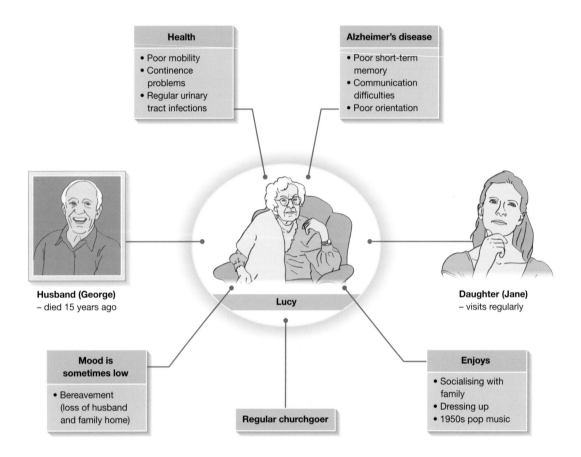

Figure 52.1 Lucy and aspects of her life, related to assessment and care plan

Health
- Poor mobility
- Continence problems
- Regular urinary tract infections

Alzheimer's disease
- Poor short-term memory
- Communication difficulties
- Poor orientation

Husband (George)
– died 15 years ago

Lucy

Daughter (Jane)
– visits regularly

Mood is sometimes low
- Bereavement (loss of husband and family home)

Regular churchgoer

Enjoys
- Socialising with family
- Dressing up
- 1950s pop music

Table 52.1 An example of part of a care plan, written with Lucy, following her initial assessment

Need or problem	Action plan	Care to be provided by	Time target
I need some help with getting to the toilet. Sometimes I do not get much warning, so I will shout. Sometimes I have infections	Nurses and carers will prompt me two-hourly during the day. They listen for my requests to go to the toilet and take me when I ask. I will tell them if I am in pain passing urine. If so, they will take a sample and ask the doctor for antibiotics if I need them	Carers and nurses	On-going
I believe in God and like to worship with other people	Carers to arrange for a minister and other people to visit me so that we can pray and sing hymns together. My daughter to take me to church once a month	Carers, the minister, my daughter	Weekly Monthly
I like to feel attractive and miss the attention of my husband	Carers will help me dress nicely and put on simple make-up. I will join in social events at the home and go out to family parties	Carers, my daughter	Daily and when arranged

Dementia Care at a Glance, First Edition. Catharine Jenkins, Laura Ginesi and Bernie Keenan. © 2016 by John Wiley & Sons, Ltd. Published 2016 by John Wiley & Sons, Ltd.
Companion website: www.ataglanceseries.com/nursing/dementiacare

The purpose of care plans

A care plan is a written record of a person's needs and the strategies they and others can use in order to address these needs. A useful and effective care plan is always based on a thorough assessment and good rapport with the person it is about. This person should be involved in defining the issues and problems addressed and have input into deciding what they want and how this should be achieved. The care plan should reflect the person's character and identity, as well as a holistic view of their needs. It is about quality of life as well as addressing problems. The care plan should be written in clear language so that any member of the team can read it quickly and follow its directions.

'I' statements

It is good practice to write the care plan together with the person with dementia and to phrase the problems identified as spoken by them, for example, 'I need help to get washed and dressed in the morning'. 'I may feel grumpy if woken too early and like a cup of tea in bed.' Similarly, solutions or 'action planning' can be written to reflect preferences, for example, 'I prefer a shower', 'I am able to carry out some parts of personal care myself and like to take my time' and 'I like to choose what to wear'. Aims, outcomes or goals should be realistic (and SMART – Specific, Measurable, Achievable, Relevant and Timely). For example, 'I will be clean and tidy and feel fresh, even if it is mid-morning'. If the person with dementia is not able to contribute to their care plan, it would be better to write it using their name, for example, 'John seems to prefer…', so that family members do not feel carers are unrealistic about the person's abilities, being untruthful or overlooking difficulties.

Crisis or emergency planning

The care plan should include emergency contact numbers and the person's wishes about what to do if they suddenly become seriously ill. Some people have an 'advance decision' stating refusal of certain care or treatment, or hospital admission in certain circumstances. The care plan should indicate where a copy of the advance decision is kept.

Incorporating biography

The care plan should reflect the person's life. Most care plans have a section for a brief life history (Chapter 39), and this can include significant events, work life, family members, likes and dislikes (Figure 52.1), significant memories, potential triggers of distress and personal effective calming measures. Family members may also be able to fill in gaps in understanding behaviour, which may be related to previous trauma, employment or relationships.

Personalising the care plan

Writing the care plan in the first person aids person-centredness (Table 52.1). The document should relate to all aspects of a person's life, not just physical and emotional needs and problems, but supportive factors as well. It should reflect aspects of identity such as cultural beliefs, sexual orientation and spirituality. The care plan is often written over a period of time, as it takes a while to build the rapport needed to support an in-depth assessment and understanding of the person. Needs will change, so the care plan should be updated regularly.

Assessment and holistic care planning

Topics to include in the care plan tend to reflect the assessment process and the main concerns of the person the plan is about and usually address issues such as:

• Physical health, including pain, long-standing conditions, mobility, sensory problems (e.g. deafness), dental health, medication
• Activities of daily living, including eating, drinking, going to the toilet, dressing
• Emotional well-being, including mood, any unusual or worrying experiences, history of mental health problems
• Communication needs and preferences
• Orientation and prompting needs
• Signs of distress and solutions that help relieve the distress
• Spiritual beliefs and expressing spirituality
• Sexuality and relationships
• Hobbies, fun and meaningful activities

Over time, people can change, and it is useful to reflect this in the person's care plan. For example, someone who has always hated spicy food may find in old age that they love curries. It is useful to communicate with families about changes to the care plan so that they can see that their relative is responded to as an individual. The nature of the care plan will differ according to the location of care and the person's life and experience of living with dementia:

• A care plan for someone living at home might have greater focus on managing risks and ensuring social inclusion.
• In a care home, the emphasis may be on personal care, comfort and reassurance.
• In hospital, standard care plans should always be personalised to reflect the needs of the individual

It is good practice to involve the person's family (with their permission) and incorporate the views of all involved in caring, so that everyone can relate to and has a sense of ownership of the plan.

Care planning for family carers

Caring can be immensely stressful and without family carers the health and social care system would be under even greater strain and financial pressure. Many aspects of caring are fulfilling, while others, for example, not being able to sleep at night, responding to aggression and faecal incontinence can be very difficult and sometimes push family members and other carers to a point where they no longer feel able to care. Therefore, it is essential to respond to the whole family's needs before individuals become desperate; it helps if they are supported so that their role is manageable and for the most part rewarding. Family members need regular time off and to share the care with others. They need information and education so that they understand the reasons for their family member's behaviour and should be aware of a range of strategies that help them cope. Carers too are individuals and depending on the person may need a listening ear, emotional support and reassurance about the care they are providing. Family members often benefit from social support and a chance to meet others in similar situations. They may feel reassured and valued if there is a contingency plan in place should they become ill themselves. They may need information about financial support and planning.

53 Personal care

Figure 53.1 Personal hygiene

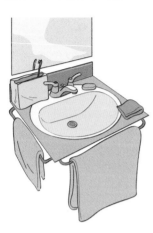

Dental care

The person should be encouraged to brush their teeth, or if they are being assisted, the carer should explain and sit in front of them at the same height and brush the back of the teeth up and down and then the front, without pushing the toothbrush too far back as this will cause them to gag. Collaboration with dental professionals will help to optimise health of people with dementia; if they wear dentures, then these need to be removed at night and soaked in a proprietary product, rinsed in clean water and brushed if necessary before reinserting. Increasingly, people have dental implants, which may require special care routines.

Washing the genitals

The person should be encouraged to wash their own genitalia, but if they cannot, when washing a male's genitalia the foreskin (if the person has one) needs to be gently retracted and the area washed, then the foreskin gently put back in place as if this is not done then constriction can occur. A female's genitalia should be washed from front to back, but not backwards and forwards in case particles from the anus are carried over the genitalia. If there is a urinary catheter, then the part of the tube that enters the body needs to be gently cleaned and dried each day to avoid residues building up.

Feet

It is important to wash in between the toes as dirt and sweat can collect there, drying thoroughly as damp areas between the toes can lead to chaffing or infection. Large emery boards are the safest way to manicure toenails, but if cutting with scissors or clippers, then cut straight across the overgrown section. Do not cut to the sides, as this can encourage in-growing toenails. If the person has circulatory problems, diabetes or toenails are very deformed or thick, then a chiropody referral should be arranged.

Figure 53.2 Providing a safe and secure environment for bathing and showering people with dementia

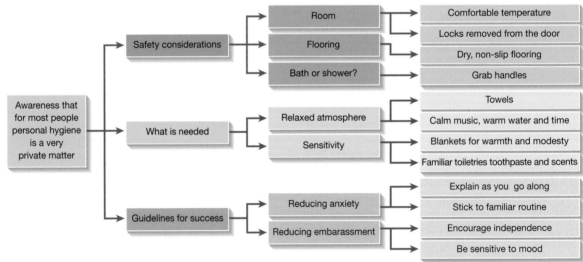

- Awareness that for most people personal hygiene is a very private matter
  - Safety considerations
    - Room
      - Comfortable temperature
      - Locks removed from the door
    - Flooring
      - Dry, non-slip flooring
    - Bath or shower?
      - Grab handles
  - What is needed
    - Relaxed atmosphere
      - Towels
      - Calm music, warm water and time
    - Sensitivity
      - Blankets for warmth and modesty
      - Familiar toiletries toothpaste and scents
  - Guidelines for success
    - Reducing anxiety
      - Explain as you go along
      - Stick to familiar routine
    - Reducing embarassment
      - Encourage independence
      - Be sensitive to mood

Figure 53.3 Personal care considerations

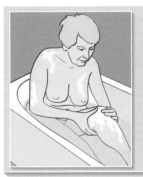

- Some people love having their hair washed, but others don't enjoy it at all. Use non-stinging shampoo and hand-held shower
- Many people do not use soap on their faces, as the skin is more sensitive
- Soap residues can damage the skin's pH balance. If using soap for the body, then it is important to rinse it off thoroughly with water
- Urinary tract infections (UTIs) are very common amongst the elderly. Genitals and the bottom should be washed every day
- Hands should be washed before eating or handling food and after using the toilet
- Try to understand how the person with dementia may be feeling and try to difuse any muddles or awkwardness by involving them in the decisions

Box 53.1 Top tip

Wash and dry throughly under folds of skin, e.g. under breasts or an overhanging paunch

Dementia Care at a Glance, First Edition. Catharine Jenkins, Laura Ginesi and Bernie Keenan. © 2016 by John Wiley & Sons, Ltd. Published 2016 by John Wiley & Sons, Ltd.
Companion website: www.ataglanceseries.com/nursing/dementiacare

Personal care

People with dementia may require help with their personal care, particularly with such tasks as washing, dressing and using the toilet. However, it is important not to assume that they will need everything to be done for them, as encouraging the individual to be as independent as possible is a vital element in maintaining their personal dignity and ability to function (Figure 53.1). Carers may sometimes feel that it is quicker to do something for the person who has dementia, but it is worth taking the time to allow them to do it for themselves so that they retain abilities.

Respect and dignity

A caring and respectful attitude towards the person with dementia contributes to an experience of respectful care that maximises dignity. Explaining what we are intending to do and asking the individual about their preferences is fundamental. Even when the person is very disorientated and they no longer understand what is being said, he/she will respond to a warm and empathetic manner, and this can be conveyed by the tone of voice, facial expression and body language (such as a relaxed open posture). Ideally a person who is known should provide care to the person with dementia; in formal care settings, the same staff should care for the person on a regular basis so that she/he becomes familiar with them. A comprehensive knowledge of the person's likes and dislikes and cultural requirements is essential; for example, an individual may not wish to be washed by somebody of a different gender, or they may prefer to wash in running water rather than static, so a shower is acceptable where a bath would not be. Alternatively, an older person who as a child only ever had a bath may feel quite frightened by a shower (Figure 53.3).

Approaches to personal care

Personal care involves an invasion of what is usually considered to be personal space and assistance with quite intimate functions, by somebody the individual may no longer recognise. This can appear to be a threatening situation or even as if the person with dementia is being assaulted, so it is not very surprising that he/she may resist personal care (Figure 53.2). There are strategies that can help (see Chapter 54), and approach and communication techniques are the most important of these. The person should be greeted by their preferred name and reminded of who the carer is, for example, 'Hello Mrs Jones, it's me, Margaret, the carer who was here yesterday'. Approaching the person who has dementia from the front is less threatening, whereas approaching quickly from behind can be frightening and may cause the person to lash out. Smiling, maintaining eye contact and conversation before and during care can help to explain what is happening and to involve the person who is being looked after in their care.

Washing and grooming

Privacy should be a priority in personal care, and although this cannot be complete if somebody needs help, carers should always try to maximise privacy, for example, by covering the person as much as possible with sheets or towels while helping them wash. Sitting upright on a chair by the bedside or at the sink in the bathroom is a much better position in which to wash than lying slumped in bed and enables the person to self-care. So wherever possible, the person should be given a bowl of water and flannels on a table in front of their bedside chair or be assisted to the bathroom to sit in front of a sink. At least two washcloths will be needed, and it is always handy to have some disposable wash cloths in case the person is incontinent. The order of washing is:

- hands and faces first
- trunk and legs
- genitalia, back and bottom

Personal preferences tend to influence this, and it is important to mimic the person's usual routines. Different washcloths should always be used for the face and the bottom and genitalia, to avoid spread of bacteria.

Dressing

Again, it is important to ensure privacy when dressing, encouraging and prompting the person with dementia to do as much for him or herself as they can. Increasing cues can also be useful, for example, laying out clothes in the order they are to be put on helps the individual with dementia avoid putting on underpants over trousers and the need for the intrusion of the carer redressing them.

Guidance on assistance with dressing

- Start with the weaker side if the person with dementia has a disability, so, for example, if they have had a 'stroke' then the affected arm would be put first into a shirt and the affected leg into the trouser.
- If dressing the upper body, place one hand under the person's elbow and another under their wrist and gently bring the arm diagonally across the body, roll the item of clothing back on your own arm first so that you can then unroll up the persons arm as you grasp their wrist, then bring it around the shoulders and move across to the other side to repeat the process of bringing the other arm into the sleeve.
- When putting on shoes, approach from the side and semi-kneel (as if proposing marriage) so that one leg can be supported on your raised knee to put the shoe on. If the person cannot extend their hip, then put the shoes on the floor and insert the feet using your thumbs to guide the heel in, but again approach from the side to avoid being accidentally kicked.

Guidance on assistance with toileting

Privacy is of course very important to everybody when using the toilet, but this has to be balanced with the help the person with dementia may need to do this in safety. If assistance onto the toilet is required, then, with the toilet immediately behind them, support the upper body with one hand by holding their shoulder, use the other hand to push down on the their hip to encourage them to bend at the hip and sit down. When using toilet paper to help people clean themselves after using the toilet, always wipe women from front to back, as this avoids particles from the anus causing infections (such as cystitis and urinary tract infections).

54 Resistance to care

Figure 54.1 Resistive behaviour

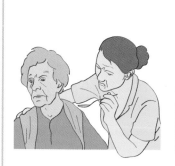
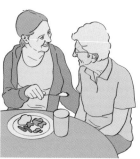
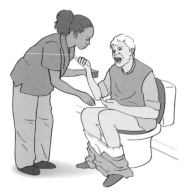
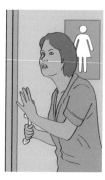

Table 54.1 Resistive behavior: possible reasons and suggested approaches

Resistive behaviour	Possible reasons	Suggested approaches
Pushing carer away during bathing or using the toilet	• Lack of understanding • Fear of exposure or loss of dignity • Feeling cold • Preference for bath or shower • Wrong time of day • Memories of childhood abuse • Pain related to restricted movement	• Ask about personal preferences and design care around them • Take a warm, sensitive approach • Consider gender of carer • Make sure to protect privacy and dignity
Refusing food	• Disliking the taste or texture • Food is not culturally appropriate • Not being orientated to time or place for eating • Not being able to see and control what is eaten • Disliking the feel of the cutlery or crockery • Toothache or poorly fitting dentures • Carers approach is not reassuring or friendly	• Ask about personal preferences and aim to meet them • Make eating a sociable experience around a dining table (if culturally appropriate) and orientate to meal time using environmental, behavioural and conversational cues • Approach from the side in a friendly, non-confrontational manner • Make encouraging comments about what the food is and how tasty it will be, e.g. "mmm chips – your favourite!"
Spitting out medication	• Fear of swallowing and choking • A horrible taste • Technique of swallowing tablets forgotten • Unclear about reason for medication	• Liaise with pharmacist about alternative formulations, e.g. better taste, medication in liquid form • Assess capacity to make the decision to refuse medication and if lacking following the principle of 'best interests' (Chapter 62) • Discuss covert medication with the person themself, family and the multi-disciplinary team
Tightly grabbing staff members arms	• Fear of falling • Grab reflex • Frustration • Protecting self from perceived assault	• Maintain the person in a position where they feel safe • Offer something else to hold, e.g. a rolled up flannel • Stroke the back of their hand to relax the fingers • Approach in a relaxed, friendly manner • Consider pain relief • Maintain dignity • Offer reassurance and distraction

Figure 54.2 Sensory perception

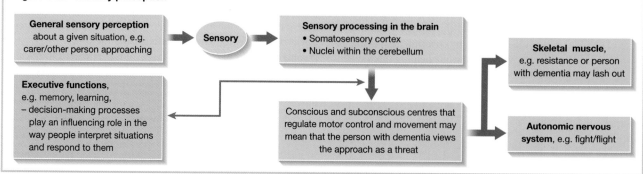

Dementia Care at a Glance, First Edition. Catharine Jenkins, Laura Ginesi and Bernie Keenan. © 2016 by John Wiley & Sons, Ltd. Published 2016 by John Wiley & Sons, Ltd.
Companion website: www.ataglanceseries.com/nursing/dementiacare

Definition

The term 'resistance to care' refers to the behaviour of a person who is unable or unwilling to cooperate with assistance and who then obstructs care either actively, for example by hitting out, or passively, by pulling away. Imagining how care might feel to someone who is disorientated and frightened can promote insight into behaviour that can be very difficult to cope with. Most resistance reflects the uncomfortable nature of personal care, which most of us would not choose even when care is at its most person-centred.

Reasons for resistance to care

People with dementia may need assistance with a range of activities of daily living. In the early stages, people are able to manage independently for the most part, but they may need help with orientation, word-finding or new technology. They may be coming to terms with their diagnosis and struggling to adjust to the future; the process involves coming to terms with loss, and a stage of this is anger (Kübler-Ross, 1969). Ordinary life stressors take more of a toll for people with dementia. They may resent attempts to protect them or comfort them. They may feel the need to fight to protect their identity, lifestyle and rights to take risks, and this can feel like irritability or rejection to family and friends. In the later stages of dementia, more help is needed with basic activities such as washing, dressing, eating and going to the toilet. It can be difficult for people with dementia to understand why other people are invading their privacy, or, as it may feel, acting towards them as if they are not competent. It also becomes more difficult for people to express themselves verbally. This is very frustrating and behaviour becomes a way of responding to stress, communicating feelings or indicating unmet needs.

Situational factors

Certain caring activities are associated with higher risk of resistance to care, and these are those associated with physical pain, such as moving from bed to chair, or emotional pain, such as feeling dignity is compromised. Using the toilet, bathing and dressing are common interactions associated with resistance. Eating, or being fed, can be difficult too. Food may not be what the person likes, or they might prefer to have it hotter or cooler. He or she may hate the way the spoon is angled or the sensation of a plastic cup against their mouth.

Environmental factors

The physical environment can aid or hinder orientation. Cues from the environment help a person understand function, for example, towels in the bathroom, salt and pepper in the dining room. If a person is unable to communicate that they are too hot or too cold, they may direct their frustration towards others in the vicinity. An environment that is crowded, noisy and too bright can be over-stimulating and stressful. The behaviour of another person with dementia can become exasperating. However, an unstimulating environment can contribute to frustration caused by boredom. Within an unsettling background, another factor can easily trigger problems.

Personal and interpersonal factors

The person-centred approach emphasises the need to know the person, their preferences and history. If a person has always had a bath, they may not recognise and feel scared by a shower. Sometimes the person with dementia may not like a carer, perhaps because of their approach or because they remind them of someone else.

Using an ABC chart to gather data on triggers

Making a record of antecedents, behaviour and consequences (ABC) gives useful information about patterns of behaviour and where it happens, who is involved, what approach was used, at what time of day it occurred and so on (Chapter 19). These trigger factors can then be adjusted so as to minimise or eradicate resistance. Listening to resistive behaviour as a form of communication can be useful. For example, if a person flexes their body to protect themselves when being washed, it could mean they have arthritic pain or are reminded of childhood abuse.

Approaches to coping

It is best to anticipate pre-empt and avoid resistance to care whenever possible, as it is harmful and stressful for both people with dementia and carers. Getting to know the person is key to providing care that suits individual needs. However, general principles can also be followed that minimise likelihood of resistance.

Communication skills

Compassion and reassurance can be communicated non-verbally. A friendly smile, a gentle tone of voice and clear, well-paced verbal and non-verbal communication allow the person to adjust to the care required. Environmental and situational cues (soap, flannel, etc.) and following personal preferences all communicate connection with the person and what the carer would like to achieve. Drawn curtains and a towel to cover the body support a sense of dignity. Friendly, natural conversation or preferred music can distract from the care process.

Pain management

Receiving care can be painful, for example, if limbs are not flexible or if a person has toothache. Prophylactic analgesia (giving painkillers in advance of a time pain may occur) means that pain is minimised and care is more comfortable. Medical and dental assessments are essential if pain is suspected. A person may not be able to tell carers about pain, but non-verbal behaviour (grimacing) and resistance (moving away, kicking or hitting) may indicate the problem.

Natural waking and personal time schedules

Sometimes resistance may be a reflection of bad timing. If a person has been woken too early, they might just need more sleep or to come round gradually and then receive personal care when they have had a cup of tea or some breakfast. Knowing the person is central; if they cannot communicate their routine, family members may be able to provide the information.

Carers' roles

Providing personal care requires excellent communication skills, emotional intelligence and physical stamina. Resistance to care can result in bruising or injury to carers. Recognition, support, training and policies to minimise harm are required to protect carers and enable them to cope with the challenging nature of their roles.

55 Sundowning syndrome and sleep

Figure 55.1 A circadian pacemaker – located in the hypothalamus – generates a rhythm that is approximately 24 hours long and which normally ensures that physiological rhythms and sleep patterns are synchronised with cycles of darkness and daylight (see Figure 55.2). The 'clock' is re-set (entrained) each day by projections from a small number of melanopsin-containing photosensitive retinal ganglion cells (PRGs)

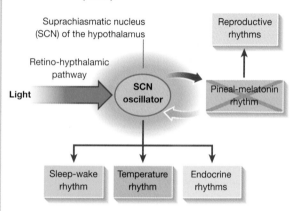

Figure 55.2 Day-Night cycle

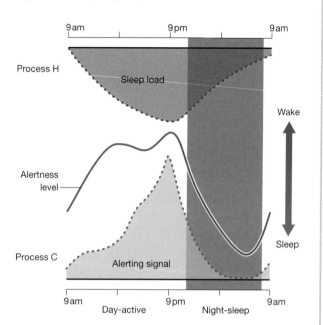

Figure 55.3 Possible triggers for 'sundowning' syndrome

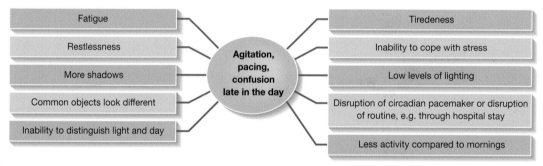

Table 55.1 Coping strategies: Responding to sundowning or disturbed sleep patterns may require trial and error, as every person is different

Comfort levels	Stress levels	Environment
• Is the person hungry, needing the toilet or in pain? • Is there something he or she needs? • Offer reassurance that everything is all right • Remind the person of the time, e.g. large analogue clock or hourglass • A doll or a pet may meet the need for comfort and connection with others	• Carry out essential tasks in the morning rather than when the person being confronted with them when least able to cope • Is enough time being allowed between activities? • Over-stimulation, e.g. noise from TV or radio causing confusion? • Are carers feeling tired and stressed? The person with dementia may pick up on it	• Avoid bathing, appointments or other potential upsetting events • Allow quiet time if it helps • Comfortable or rocking chair may provide gentle stimulation • Aromatherapy, e.g. lavender oil, chamomile, bergamot may have calming effect and reduce agitation
Light levels and shadows • Improve levels of lighting during daylight hours • Sit outdoors in daylight hours if weather allows • Use night lights • Leave a door open to hallways	**Managing disorientation** • Make sure doors are external doors are locked to prevent a disorientated person from walking outside • Provide reassurance if the person is having difficulty separating dreams from reality when sleeping • Avoid contradicting the person or arguing, as this may confuse and distress everyone	**Evening routines** • Close curtains and lower light levels when darkness falls each evening • Play favourite music and provide familiar objects to reassure • Ensure there are no hazards • Door sensors and safety gates can alert family members to wandering
Sleep hygiene • Avoid stimulants (caffeine, sweets, nicotine) and large dinners and alcohol in the evenings • Anti-psychotics, sedatives, melatonin may help some people • Avoid physical activity in 3–4 hours before bedtime • Encourage a regular bedtime routine	**Activity levels** • Brisk walks or outings during the day may reduce need to wander later • Group games, dancing, resistance training, etc. can improve mood and lift spirits • Setting the table or helping with meal preparations can help to distract the person with dementia	**Physical ailments may include** • Urinary tract infections • Incontinence problems • Restless leg syndrome • Sleep apnoea (abnormal breathing pattern where people briefly stop breathing many times a night)

Dementia Care at a Glance, First Edition. Catharine Jenkins, Laura Ginesi and Bernie Keenan. © 2016 by John Wiley & Sons, Ltd. Published 2016 by John Wiley & Sons, Ltd.
Companion website: www.ataglanceseries.com/nursing/dementiacare

Human circadian clocks are the body's genetically determined cycles of molecular, cellular, physiological, emotional and behavioural patterns (Figure 55.1). Some people are 'larks' who tend to feel more active and alert in the morning, while others are 'owls' who have a later to bed, later to rise body type. Morningness or eveningness traits, therefore, influence when people prefer to eat, exercise, make love and many other activities.

Drivers of sleep-wakefulness

Sleep is a complex behaviour that is an integral part of our adaptation to daily changes in light and temperature and recent research is transforming understanding of the process of sleep and the way it arises from a network of activity in the brain.

Sleep is regulated by two key opposing systems (Figure 55.2):

- **Process C:** a spontaneously generated internal 24-hour circadian rhythm of sleep and arousal determined by a physiological 'clock' located in the suprachiasmatic nuclei (SCN) of the hypothalamus.
- **Process H:** a homeostatic 'counter' that responds to sleep pressure. The longer you have been awake, the greater the level of sleep pressure or need to sleep. During sleep, the level of sleep pressure falls until we wake up.

These circadian and homeostatic processes regulate multiple brain circuits to synchronise physiological functions at systems and organ level. Drowsiness (or **sleep induction**) appears to be driven by an inhibitory 'switch' – a group of GABA-ergic neurons in the ventrolateral preoptic (VLPO) nucleus of the hypothalamus is active while we sleep and inhibits arousal patterns. Neurons in the brainstem produce monoamine neurotransmitters (noradrenaline, histamine, dopamine and serotonin) that keep some parts of the brain active while we are awake. In turn, these neurons are activated by orexin-producing neurons in the hypothalamus that are important for eating behaviours and hunger.

Sleep architecture

There are two distinct kinds of sleep, and adults have four to five alternating cycles of rapid eye movement (REM) sleep and non-rapid eye movement (NREM) sleep during an average night although proportions of each type of NREM and REM in each cycle changes throughout the night.

Both types of sleep are characterised by orderly patterns of electrical activity that can be recorded using electroencephalogram (EEG), electromyogram (EMG), electro-oculogram (EOG) and other physiological measures:

- REM sleep is sometimes called 'paradoxical sleep' because there is increased heart rate, irregular, shallower breathing, poor temperature control, higher blood pressure and improved cerebral blood flow accompanied by inhibition of skeletal muscle activity (atonia). EEG patterns during this phase are almost identical to those of a person who is awake.
- NREM sleep generally associated with more stable physiological measures, for example, more regular breathing and lower heart rate. Memory consolidation and movement take place whilst conscious awareness of the external world disappears.

Sleep in the elderly

A good night's sleep isn't just refreshing; an individual's chronotype reflects the time of day physiological functions including hormone levels, body temperature, cognitive skills, eating patterns and sleeping patterns are at their most active. Sleep **quotas** refer to the relative amount of time spend in REM or NREM sleep, while **phasing** describes the way sleep is distributed over a 24-hour period.

Humans' need for sleep appears to be constant, but elderly people often report that they find it harder to fall asleep and to stay asleep; they seem to spend more time in the lighter stages of sleep than in deep sleep and awakenings seem to increase.

These shifting patterns have been associated with changes in the SCN pacemaker that disrupts the way process C and process H interact with each other. Some older people have diminished capacity to produce melatonin, which may further limit the duration of sleep. It may be that people sleep less as they get older because of a gradual reduction in the number of VLPO neurons that turn off arousal systems. However, age-related changes, including poorer circulation, temperature regulation, cataracts and macular degeneration, have also been implicated.

Dementia

Improved knowledge of circadian rhythms (and consideration of factors identified in Figure 55.3) can thus help to explain the 'sundowning' syndrome – the way in which people with dementia may become more restless, confused, agitated, aggressive, unusually demanding and/or active in the late afternoon and evening. Dementia also exacerbates disturbances in sleep–wake patterns, and night-time wakening is strongly related to cognitive and functional decline.

Dementia leads to disruption to circadian rhythms and deterioration of neurons in the SCN 'master clock'. Eventually, many people with dementia may lose track of time and forget when they last ate, when bedtime is, accuse carers of having been away for hours, become frightened at night and so on. This kind of disruption can be extremely challenging for caregivers to deal with and is a common cause of institutionalisation of older people who have dementia.

Light and circadian rhythms

Although driven by the body's networks of timekeepers, these rhythms must be reset every day to ensure that they are synchronised with the external environment. In normal circumstances, light exposure is the primary cue (or *zeitgeber*) that entrains the many internal clocks of the human body. Photosensitive ganglion cells in the retina (pRCGs) project to the SCN (see Figure 55.1) and provide information about ambient light levels and day length. Light exposure inhibits secretion of melatonin – the 'sleepiness' hormone – from the pineal gland (Figure 55.1) and has mood-enhancing and anti-depressant effects.

People with dementia do not always get outside every day and may take more daytime 'naps', so there is potential for reinforcing light – dark cycles by improving levels of light that may make sleep cycles more robust (see Table 55.1).

56 Transitions

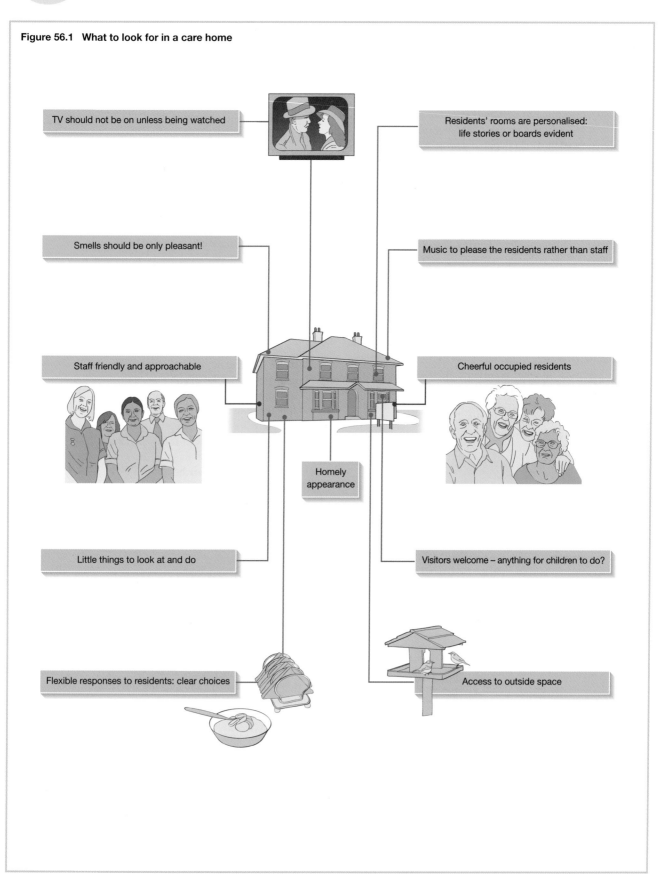

Figure 56.1 What to look for in a care home

TV should not be on unless being watched

Residents' rooms are personalised: life stories or boards evident

Smells should be only pleasant!

Music to please the residents rather than staff

Staff friendly and approachable

Cheerful occupied residents

Homely appearance

Little things to look at and do

Visitors welcome – anything for children to do?

Flexible responses to residents: clear choices

Access to outside space

Dementia Care at a Glance, First Edition. Catharine Jenkins, Laura Ginesi and Bernie Keenan. © 2016 by John Wiley & Sons, Ltd. Published 2016 by John Wiley & Sons, Ltd.
Companion website: www.ataglanceseries.com/nursing/dementiacare

Reasons for relocation

A diagnosis of dementia does not mean a person is no longer safe to live alone or that they need supervision. Most people with dementia continue to live fulfilling lives in their own homes, making adjustments as necessary to ensure their condition does not lead to risks. The risks that may occur and potential solutions are given below.

Risks	Solutions
Forgetting the key and being locked out	Leave a key with a neighbour.
Leaving the gas on	Arranging a gas alarm, automatic cut off or controlled access to gas. It may be possible to disconnect gas appliances and change over to easy to use electrical alternatives.
Dishonest people taking advantage	Have a chain link on the door and notices on the window stating no callers. Ask a family member to take out a lasting power of attorney (LPA) for finances (Chapter 62), and to monitor for concerning patterns. Let local police and neighbours know so that they can keep an eye out.
Self-neglect, for example not eating or washing adequately	Arrange a home care and meals on wheels service, via local social services or privately
Frequent falls	Wear a fall detector that alerts a family member, friend or neighbour who could call over and investigate

Issues related to mental capacity

While the risks listed above naturally lead to concern, if the person with dementia is able to understand and accept these risks and adjustments, preferring them to life in different accommodation, then they have the right to do so. If the behaviour of the person with dementia is causing risks to others, for example, if gas leaks could result in an explosion or if they regularly wander in the road and could cause an accident, then it is possible that they do not have capacity to make the decision (this should be assessed) and a solution that supports their well-being should be sought, in their best interests while being the least restrictive option (Chapter 62). A package of care within which regular carers visits are arranged to meet the person's needs, complemented by assistive technology (Chapter 44) to promote safety is a positive alternative if agreed by the person with dementia.

Positive choices

Living alone can be lonely and isolating, and for many people the decision to move to be either nearer to or with family, or into a care home, is a positive one. For some the decision is prompted out of concern for the well-being of a carer. Forward planning (an advance statement) enables the person with memory problems to take part in choosing their new home and to retain an important degree of autonomy. If considering residential or nursing home care, it is usually possible to go for respite care or a trial visit. The person with dementia should be encouraged to write down their feelings about the home (or a family member could film them using a mobile phone while talking about it) so that they can use this information later in deciding what to do. Occasionally a care package can become very expensive, meaning that a care home is financially beneficial.

Triggers for unplanned relocations

Deterioration in the person with dementia's condition, a serious health problem, or symptoms that cause unmanageable stress or distress for family carers can be implicated in unplanned transitions. A hospital stay may be essential for assessment and management of another health issue but could have a negative impact on the person's orientation and functioning. Admissions should be as brief as possible and every support given to enable the person to remain self-caring. The toilet should be visible from the bed and continence prioritised, as being continent is a significant factor in a successful discharge home. Carers should receive practical and psychological support so that the pressure does not become overwhelming (Chapter 48). Regular respite care makes a transition later less traumatic for both the person with dementia and the family carer.

Avoiding relocation

Relocations often involve difficult adjustments that are exacerbated for people with dementia because of the additional disorientation and problems remembering the reasons for the move. A move may be essential, but limiting the number of moves will be beneficial, so it is better to use strategies that minimise the need for relocations, while managing them effectively when necessary.

Strategies to reduce the need for relocation

- Minimise risks, as outlined earlier
- Maximise orientation – keep the same or similar colours around the home, reinforce a daily routine (Chapter 45)
- Every person should have access to their own possessions, clothing, money, handbag, etc.
- Use glasses or hearing aids if they are needed
- Maintain physical health through a good diet, exercise and managing any health problems
- Design a personalised care plan and employ trusted carers to carry it out
- Use assistive technology (Chapter 44) to prompt with medication, alert to risks (e.g. doors open, gas left on, water overflowing)
- Put prompts around the house, for example, reminders on the back door not to forget keys
- Carry a card with name address and next of kin for emergency contact in case of accident or becoming lost
- Include the person in family life so that they do not feel lonely

Choosing a care home

The person with dementia should be involved in decision-making as far as possible. His or her priorities should be borne in mind and choices respected. If it is clear that permanent care will be needed, it is best to plan so that only one move is needed, and the person might choose a home where a range of care requirements can be met. The person with dementia should also consider who they would like to be able to visit them and how easy this will be. They may need to think about whether their pet can move with them (Chapter 43), if there is an accessible garden and what activities they can take part in (Chapter 35). In choosing a care home the person and their family could look at Care Quality Commission (CQC) inspection reports online, visit a range of homes and see where they felt most comfortable (see Figure 56.1). The welcome friendliness and caring qualities of staff, and the relationships between staff, will have the greatest impact on quality of life of those for whom they care.

57 Walking

Figure 57.1 Reasons for walking

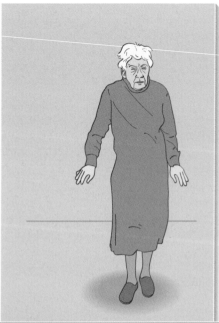

Reasons for walking	Strategy to meet unmet need
The person may:	**Staff can:**
• Need to use the toilet	• Show the person the way to the toilet and assist if necessary
• Be tired and be looking for their bedroom	• Direct them to their bed and assist if necessary
• Be in pain but unable to express this	• Give analgesia and observe for effects on mood and behaviour
• Be hungry or thirsty and looking for something to eat or drink	• Offer food and drink
• Be bored or frightened	• Reassure, spend time with the person
• Be seeking a loved one or their own home	• Reassure, re-orientate, explain, spend time
• Be reliving the past and still performing the duties attached to their previous occupation, e.g. as a postman	• Redirect so that the walking does not impact negatively on others
• Be looking for a landmark	• Point out landmarks, consider providing additional landmarks and signage in the environment
• Have always enjoyed physical activity which includes long walks, and they are simply attempting to continue their normal routine	• Discuss with person and family, try to include walking opportunities in daily routine

Box 57.1 Top tips

- Reframe 'wandering' as communication of unmet needs or a positive healthy activity

- Identify and meet any unmet needs

- Maintain safety – encourage the person to walk in areas where they are not posing a risk to themselves or others

If a person is at risk when walking outside, then they should be:

- Dressed in warm clothes to minimise the risk of hypothermia

- Wearing shoes with a good grip and have their walking aid to hand to help prevent falls

- Carrying some form of identification, whether an identification band on their wrist or a piece of paper in their pocket stating their name and address

Dementia Care at a Glance, First Edition. Catharine Jenkins, Laura Ginesi and Bernie Keenan. © 2016 by John Wiley & Sons, Ltd. Published 2016 by John Wiley & Sons, Ltd.
Companion website: www.ataglanceseries.com/nursing/dementiacare

Walking is healthy

There are many reasons why a person with dementia may choose or wish to walk about and these reasons are usually logical, although they may not always be obvious to other people (Figure 57.1). As walking is a healthy activity, it should be encouraged and if the current pattern of a person's walking is creating risk, it is better to aim to redirect their walking rather than to stop it. Sometimes walking can be identified as a problem, for example, if the person with dementia leaves their home to go to the shops and then gets lost or if they are on a busy hospital ward and go into other patients' rooms. The term 'wandering' is sometimes used, but this can stigmatise and undermine the person, while not addressing their needs. If the walking is creating a risk for the person and difficulties for others, it is better to aim to understand the underlying reasons and then to address them.

Promoting safe walking

Assistive technology, for example, movement-activated lighting, such as floor sensors, can help avoid falls if the person with dementia gets up to walk about during the night (see chapters on falls and assistive technology). Alarms can alert carers to the person moving or exiting the area.

Many purpose-built spaces now include a circular or 'circuit' corridor where people with dementia can safely enjoy a lengthy walk. Some of these now incorporate 'activity' stations with a variety of objects placed to engage and occupy the people walking there.

Secure garden areas with non-slip flooring and somewhere safe to sit enable the person with dementia to continue to enjoy being outdoors. It not only allows the individual to engage in activity that they may always have valued but also maximises the health-related benefits of access to the available sunlight and fresh air.

Problematic walking or 'wandering'

If the person with dementia is living at home and often goes out and gets lost and is at risk when crossing the road, or of being out in the cold at night, or in danger of being taken advantage of by other people, family members and neighbours naturally become worried. The Dementia Friendly Communities Initiative (UK) is designed partly to raise awareness and encourage the public to be more supportive and helpful in these situations (Chapter 30). Assistive technology can be very useful and aid the person to manage these risks and continue to live in their own home (Chapter 44). Personal trackers can be worn; they use satellite technology and ensure the person can always be found. A door alert that activates when the front door is opened and plays a message recorded by a family member such as 'Stay home Dad, it's dark now' can be effective. If the reason for going out is to seek company, local voluntary organisations may be able to offer a befriending service.

If the person with dementia is in a hospital or care environment, problems tend to arise when a person's walking interferes with the needs of other patients (e.g. if the walking person keeps going near medical equipment and may inadvertently adjust it) or when other residents need to relax and have privacy. Distraction and alternative activities are useful in these situations, so knowing the person and their interests is useful, so as to tap into those interests. If a member of staff needs to go on an errand, it can be useful for them to be accompanied by the person who likes to walk.

Excessive walking as an indication of unmet need

Behaviour always has a reason and walking without an obvious purpose can be an expression of a person looking for something or somebody, or of feeling bored, or being physically uncomfortable.

Orientation

Regular reorientation, explaining to the person with dementia where they are, what is happening and who is looking after them can make them feel safe. For the person who is repeatedly looking for their relatives, it can be helpful to have a written message from the loved one explaining where they are and when the relative will next visit. (Please see Chapter 50 for difficult conversations when they are looking for a loved one who has died.) A visible clock is known to help with orientation, as is a prominently placed whiteboard with details of the date and location (Chapter 40).

Good lighting and minimising background noise can reduce agitation while increasing cues by having large pictorial signs on doors can help prevent the person feeling or actually getting lost.

If boredom is the cause, something interesting to do and friendly people to chat with can make the person more likely to stay.

Others affected by a person's walking may need reassurance, for example, in a hospital staff can 'model' a calm approach to redirecting the person.

Restraint

Use of sedation or confining by locking doors should always be a last resort. 'Passive restraints' can offer a more humane alternative to maintaining the person's safety. These can include:

- Baffle handles and digital locks
- Doors painted in the same colour as the surrounding walls to make them less obvious

On-going health benefits of walking

Regular walking may slow the progression of dementia. It also reduces frustration and boosts mood. We all need exercise to remain healthy and happy, and the person with dementia will benefit through enjoying company, using some energy and being active and occupied.

58 End-of-life care

Table 58.1   The PAINAD pain assessment in (people with) advanced dementia scale

Indicator	Score = 0	Score = 1	Score = 2	Total score
Breathing	• Normal breathing	• Occasional laboured breathing • Short period of hyperventilation	• Noisy laboured breathing • Long period of hyperventilation • Cheyne-Stokes respiration	
Negative vocalisations	• None	• Occasional moan/groan • Low level, speech with a negative or disapproving quality	• Repeated troubled calling out • Loud moaning or groaning • Crying	
Facial expression	• Smiling or inexpressive	• Sad, frightened, frown	• Facial grimace	
Body language	• Relaxed	• Tense, distressed, pacing, fidgeting	• Rigid, fists clenched • Knees pulled up • Striking out • Pulling or pushing away	
Consolability	• No need to console	• Distracted by voice or touch	• Unable to console, distract or reassure	

The score ranges from 0 – no pain to 10 – severe pain   **Total:**

Source: *Warden V, Hurley AC & Volicer L. Journal of the American Medical Directors Association 2003; 4(1); 9-15. Reproduced with permission of Elsevier*

Box 58.1   'Sinking'

Tap drips
A metronome
Time leaks away
along with bits of me–
toenails, hair, skin,
memories drain
out to the grey sea

Source: *Reproduced by permission of Sue Carroll*

Figure 58.1   The World Health Organisation Pain Relief Ladder

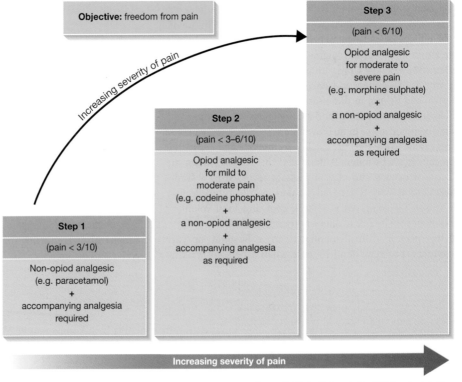

Source: *World Health Organisation (WHO) analgesic ladder*

Dementia Care at a Glance, First Edition. Catharine Jenkins, Laura Ginesi and Bernie Keenan. © 2016 by John Wiley & Sons, Ltd. Published 2016 by John Wiley & Sons, Ltd.
Companion website: www.ataglanceseries.com/nursing/dementiacare

Issues around death and dying

Death is a normal process in life—we all die. As our body systems age, we will often develop a multitude of physical problems, so people with dementia may die from completely unrelated conditions, such as cardiac problems or cancer. Dementia, however, is ultimately a terminal illness; people with dementia can often lose the ability to swallow and cough properly as the condition progresses, thus becoming more prone to dehydration, kidney failure and chest infections as a cause of death. Whatever the reason for the terminal illness, the emphasis should always be on enhancing the quality of life and involving people with dementia and those who care for them in the planning of their care. In the community, this will be coordinated by the GP, community nurses and palliative care teams.

The Leadership Alliance for the Care of Dying People (2014) has drawn up five key priorities for care:

- Recognition that death is imminent
- Communicating sensitively with the person and their family regarding this
- Involving them in decisions
- Supporting them and their family
- Creating an individual plan of care that is delivered with compassion and that involves adequate nutrition and hydration

End-of-life care or palliative care is not about hastening or postponing death; it is about offering support to help people live as actively and comfortably as possible and to avoid unnecessary hospital admissions. Most people would prefer to die in their own homes, but this is not always possible because carers cannot always cope with the increased needs for physical care or behavioural changes. Additionally, hospice places are not always available and rely on a definitive time scale for death, which is often not possible for people with dementia. If a transition to residential care or hospital is required, then the person should be supported by frequent visits from loved ones.

Advance care planning

The person with dementia may want to clarify their wishes for their end-of-life care. An 'advance decision' relates to treatment the person would like to refuse, for example, artificial feeding. This is a written and formally witnessed statement made when they are deemed to have capacity and is legally enforceable (Chapter 62). An 'advance statement' relates to the care and treatment that the person would prefer. This is less formal and can be spoken or written. Considering end-of-life issues encourages communication between all involved, promotes individuals' autonomy and can provide guidance on care and treatment when the person is no longer able to voice their wishes.

Spiritual issues

The concept of 'choice' for the person who is dying incorporates the need to make individual preparations for death that include not only choice about where to die and the interventions that may be used at that time but also time to settle their financial and spiritual affairs. Spirituality is a very individual concept (Chapter 17) and can mean psychological acceptance of death, for which counselling services can be helpful. Spirituality also encompasses the religious or cultural rituals that are important for the person to feel at peace. Talking about death and dying can be difficult; family members may need support and access to bereavement counselling.

Comfort and dignity

People with dementia do not always volunteer that they are experiencing pain, so carers need to be proactive about asking them to self-rate pain, for example, by the use of a visual analogue scale such as the common Faces Pain Scale. However, people who are in the late stages of dementia may be unable to communicate their needs, so carers need to be observant for signs of pain or distress, including grimacing, rubbing, restlessness, pacing, agitation or aggression. The Pain Assessment in Advanced Dementia Scale (PAINAD) assists with assessment of pain using non-verbal indicators (Table 58.1). Knowing the person comprehensively, their known ailments, and normal behaviour is also a great help in recognising the likelihood of pain and anticipating for this with prophylactic analgesia. If there are indications of pain, then analgesia should always be given and reviewed for effectiveness. Generally speaking, the mildest analgesics will be used first and the type and amount increased as required (see Figure 58.1). Non-pharmacological interventions can also help, for example, hot or cold pads, repositioning, elevating swollen limbs and massage.

Swallowing may become more difficult in the latter stages of dementia, which raises problems of maintaining adequate hydration, particularly if the person is deemed to be at risk of inhaling the liquids they are drinking. Unfortunately this can often result in hospital admission and requests for artificial nutrition and hydration such as intravenous fluids (a 'drip') or nasogastric feeds (via a tube between nose and stomach). Invasive treatments such as these may prolong life but not contribute to a dignified death. Other methods can be used in the person's own environment to maintain comfort, such as keeping the lips and mouth moist, or minimally invasive procedures such as using a subcutaneous infusion with a small amount of liquid going into the body under the skin. An assessment by a speech and language therapist (SALT) can also result in alternative methods such as thickened fluids that are more easily swallowed.

'Do not resuscitate' orders

Euthanasia is illegal in the United Kingdom, but there may be instances when a hospital physician or GP may recommend that no unnecessary measures be taken to prolong the life of a person who is terminally ill or dying. 'Do not resuscitate' decisions are made on the basis of the wishes of the person, opinions of family members, the likelihood of success of the proposed interventions and the quality of life that could be achieved for the individual. Decisions relate to such issues as not using of basic life support procedures and defibrillation if a person's heart stopped beating, and not treating infections with antibiotics. However, emergency measures would still be used if, for example, the person were choking. The 'do not resuscitate' decision must be in writing and signed by a doctor to be valid; it is a legal requirement that the person and their family are aware of these decisions.

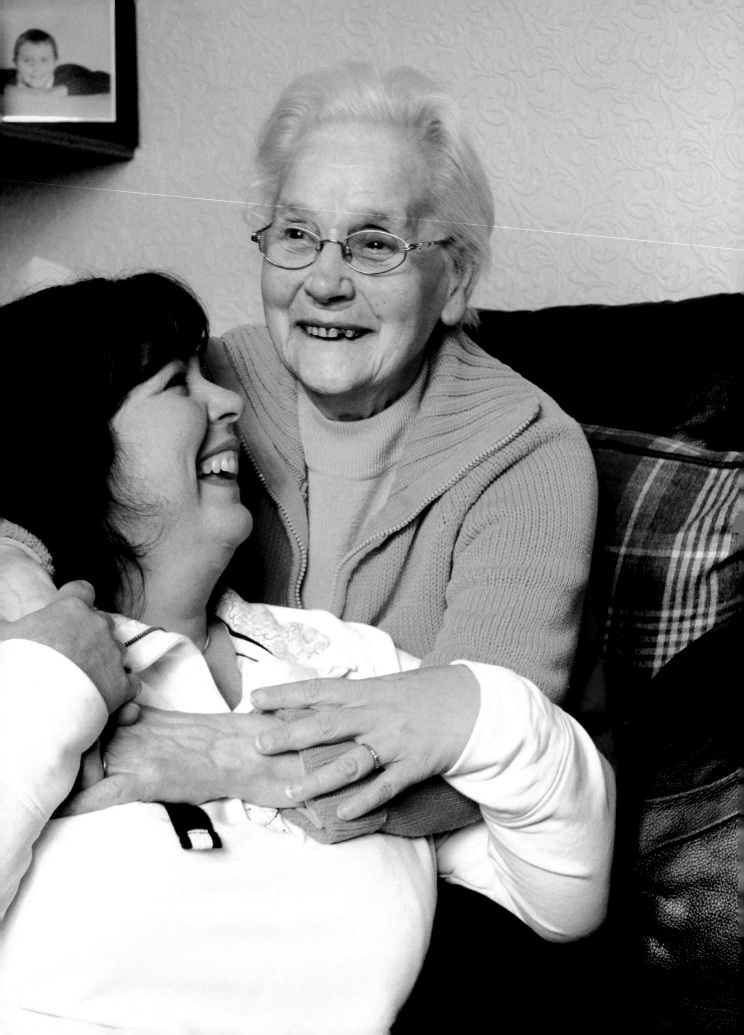

Ethical and legal issues

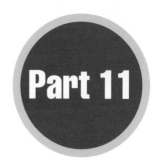

Part 11

Chapters

59 Abuse, neglect and safeguarding

Figure 59.1 Signs of abuse

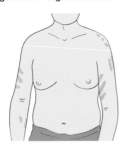

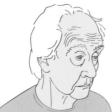

Indicators of physical abuse

Bruises, bite marks, lacerations, cigarette burns, finger marks, broken teeth, hair loss, weight loss, marks in the shape of objects, and repeated bruising or injuries. If inappropriately sedated, the person will appear to be very drowsy or sleep excessively.

Indicators of psychological abuse

Depression or withdrawal, anxiety, self- harm, overly compliant behaviour, loss of appetite, insomnia. The person with dementia may be anxious or fearful, or have sudden change in known behaviour (e.g. suddenly aggressive). Carers may also be alerted by overly controlling or critical behaviour on the part of someone connected with the vulnerable person.

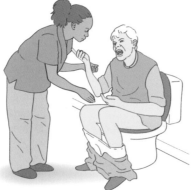

Indicators of sexual abuse

Anal/genital bleeding or bruising or tearing, persistent vulval reddening or discharge, sexually transmitted diseases. The person may experience discomfort or difficulty walking or sitting or may display, reluctance to remove underwear in situations of supervised bathing.

Overtly sexualised behaviour, self-harm/genital mutilation.

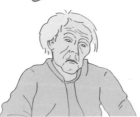

Indicators of neglect

Dehydration, malnutrition, poor hygiene, pressure sores, inadequate clothing, untreated medical conditions, loneliness and distress are possible signs of neglect.

There may be a noticeable loss of weight but the person concerned could have a voracious appetite when they are offered food.

Indicators of financial abuse

Deterioration in living standards, inability to pay bills or buy essentials, where the individual does not have the lifestyle that reflects their income, loss of money or unexplained withdrawals from accounts, uncertain signatures on documents, sudden or unexplained transfer of property, care homes that cannot produce financial records for clients.

Box 59.1 Top tips

- Be alert to the indicators of abuse

- Document your concerns in a permanent record

- Report immediately to social care and health or a designated safeguarding team if there is one

- Preserve any evidence

- Alert the police if you feel that a crime has been committed

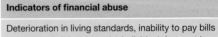

Dementia Care at a Glance, First Edition. Catharine Jenkins, Laura Ginesi and Bernie Keenan. © 2016 by John Wiley & Sons, Ltd. Published 2016 by John Wiley & Sons, Ltd.
Companion website: www.ataglanceseries.com/nursing/dementiacare

The vast majority of older people with dementia are not abused or neglected, but when it happens and is reported by the media, the outcry and concerns raised lead to fears that unacceptable behaviour towards people with dementia is widespread. Nevertheless, abuse does occasionally occur and may range on a continuum from disrespectful language to serious physical harm. People with dementia may be particularly open to abuse because the nature of their condition can give rise to huge stress among caregivers. The person with dementia may be dependent on others to manage their financial resources, because caregivers and the looked after person may be isolated and under-supported and because perpetrators may think a person with dementia will forget or not be believed. Most people with dementia are physically unable to run away or fight back. Under-valuing belief systems (e.g. a person with dementia is no longer a full citizen) may lead others into feeling that abuse towards them is less serious than it would be to a child or mentally competent adult.

Abuse

Abuse is any violation of an individual's human or civil rights by any other person or persons. Abuse is not caused by the vulnerability of the older person but by other people's responses to it. There are certain circumstances that make abuse more likely:

• Alcohol abuse by a carer
• Poor mental health of a carer
• Carer and person with dementia isolated and unsupported
• A family pattern of violence
• Previous abuse by the person with dementia of the carer, for example, child abuse
• The carer is in some way (e.g. financially) dependent on the person they look after
• Paid carers who are themselves poorly treated by employers and as a consequence feel powerless, yet are in positions of power over their residents or patients

Despite the stressors of working in dementia care, most carers find the role rewarding and commit themselves to promoting the well-being of their family member or service user.

Safeguarding

Safeguarding is the term used to refer to the protection of vulnerable people from abuse, neglect, discrimination, embarrassment or poor treatment. The Human Rights Act (1998) addresses the right of every adult to live in safety, free from the fear of possible abuse from others. Keeping people safe does not mean preventing vulnerable adults from leading an independent life – which inevitably contains elements of risk – but is about minimising those risks where possible.

Abusers

Abusers can be both male and female, family members or paid carers and lone abusers or groups. Abuse transcends class and cultural boundaries. The abuse can constitute single or repeated acts.

Poor practice

An environment that dehumanises the person with dementia by providing substandard care or by belittling, objectifying or infantilising them can create a culture where abuse is more likely.

Poor practice should therefore be challenged, and those providing it should be guided so that they improve the care offered.

Types of abuse

• **Physical abuse**: punching, kicking, biting, slapping, burning, cutting, torture, inappropriate use of medication, inappropriate manual handling and domestic abuse. This can also incorporate the use of unlawful chemical or physical restraints
• **Sexual abuse**: any sexual act to which the person does not or cannot consent, for example, rape, sexual assault, sex trafficking, forced marriage and domestic abuse
• **Financial abuse**: fraud, theft, embezzlement, exploitation, or coercion to part with goods/services/property and misappropriation of money/goods/property
• **Psychological abuse**: bullying, threatening, humiliation, insulting, blaming, controlling, denying privacy, harassment, isolation, abandonment, and domestic abuse
• **Neglect**: ignoring physical or care needs, starvation, abandonment, failure to provide necessary access to services, withholding of essential items, for example, heating or bedding or medication
• **Discriminatory abuse**: actions targeted at individuals because of race or ethnic grouping, religion, gender, sexual orientation or because they have a learning disability (including 'mate hate').
• **Institutional abuse**: inappropriate behaviours or care occurring in a formal care setting, which can consist of many of the various different types of abuse already mentioned. Any restrictions or restraints in an institutional setting require formal documentation and independent monitoring under the Deprivation of Liberty Safeguards (DoLS) as required by the Mental Capacity Act (2005). If this does not happen, it can be classified as institutional abuse

If abuse occurs

If a professional or family member notices indications of abuse as in Figure 59.1, or a person with dementia reports abuse, it is important to take it seriously and report it to the appropriate authority. It is better to escalate a false allegation than to leave a vulnerable person open to further abuse; however, recording and reporting concerns accurately should protect both the person with dementia and alleged perpetrator. Abuse in any setting should be reported immediately to the local safeguarding team/ social care and health office.

Advice on tackling abuse

• Do not put yourself or anyone else in danger.
• Discuss concerns with a service manager, local safeguarding team or local social care and health personnel.
• Document the problems in a factual, non-judgemental way.
• Do not accuse anyone of abuse, as this may be viewed as libel, just state exactly what you have seen or heard, using quotation marks to note anything you have been told.
• Professionals should always document in a permanent client record.
• Most local guidelines call for safeguarding referral within 12 hours of the concerns being raised. It is not obligatory to get permission from the suspected victim or the suspected perpetrator to refer, although it is good practice to inform them of the referral unless it is felt that this would put the abused person in more danger.
• Preserve any evidence of abuse.
• Inform the police if you feel that a crime has been committed, for example, physical assault, sexual assault theft or fraud.

60 Ethical issues

Figure 60.1 Conflicting needs and thoughts

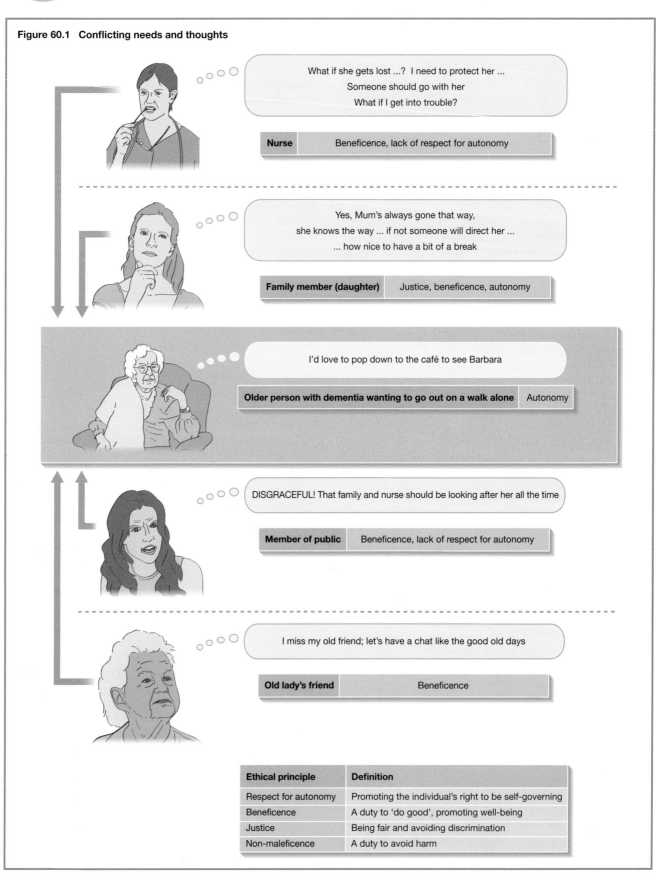

What if she gets lost ...? I need to protect her ...
Someone should go with her
What if I get into trouble?

| Nurse | Beneficence, lack of respect for autonomy |

Yes, Mum's always gone that way,
she knows the way ... if not someone will direct her ...
... how nice to have a bit of a break

| Family member (daughter) | Justice, beneficence, autonomy |

I'd love to pop down to the café to see Barbara

| Older person with dementia wanting to go out on a walk alone | Autonomy |

DISGRACEFUL! That family and nurse should be looking after her all the time

| Member of public | Beneficence, lack of respect for autonomy |

I miss my old friend; let's have a chat like the good old days

| Old lady's friend | Beneficence |

Ethical principle	Definition
Respect for autonomy	Promoting the individual's right to be self-governing
Beneficence	A duty to 'do good', promoting well-being
Justice	Being fair and avoiding discrimination
Non-maleficence	A duty to avoid harm

Dementia Care at a Glance, First Edition. Catharine Jenkins, Laura Ginesi and Bernie Keenan. © 2016 by John Wiley & Sons, Ltd. Published 2016 by John Wiley & Sons, Ltd.
Companion website: www.ataglanceseries.com/nursing/dementiacare

Ethical principles

The purpose of ethical principles is to guide people about what is right and what is wrong. This can be difficult to decide in the field of dementia care because there are often clashes of interest, so that for example what is right for the person with dementia may not be right for others, for example, a family carer (Figure 60.1). Sometimes the interests of the person with dementia are difficult to identify, for example at times they may need to be protected while at other times need to assert their own wishes. Ethical principles provide a structure and language to aid discussion of the moral quandaries that can arise. These principles are:

- Respect for autonomy
- Beneficence
- Non-maleficence
- Justice

Truthfulness and fairness are sometimes added to this list.

Ethical dilemmas

A dilemma involves a decision that needs to be made, but where each option has equal or similar (usually negative) outcomes. This makes decision-making difficult. Dilemmas involving people with dementia usually have an ethical component because the person with dementia may be perceived as vulnerable and needing protection, but they are also adults with views and desires that should be respected. Thus, a common clash occurs between the duty to do good (beneficence) and respect for autonomy.

Autonomy

Dementia is a progressive condition that gradually harms the capacity to weigh up complex arguments. It also damages communication skills and the ability to carry out a sequence of activities, all of which are needed for autonomous functioning. In Western culture, there is an assumption that each individual makes decisions independently, but this is not reflected in reality, most people across the world are part of inter-dependent networks of family and friends. For the person with dementia, there is often a gradual transition from an independent or inter-dependent existence towards acceptance that other people will take care of major decision-making. This transition may lead to distress and conflict, so the person with dementia will need support and understanding.

Driving a car

The car is both a means of getting about and a symbol of independence. Being able to drive is a marker of adulthood, and for many their car is chosen to reflect status. Driving is not prohibited for people with a diagnosis of dementia; in the early stages, most people can continue to drive safely. However, it is a legal requirement in most countries to report a diagnosis and to have regular driving assessments. Therefore, it is obvious that this most valuable capability is threatened. To take away a person's driving licence (and maybe their car) is often a huge blow, affecting self-esteem as well as limiting lifestyle. On the other hand, the risk to others if a person's driving becomes unsafe is clearly unacceptable. Society as a whole and the person with dementia have to balance the conflicting needs of protecting the public with maintaining a person's (or couples') autonomy. Use of public transportation or taxis can save money, be more sociable and less stressful, alternatively a lift rota could be created by friends and family.

Duty of care and positive risk-taking

Health and social care professionals are bound by codes of conduct that emphasise commitment to the welfare of others, sometimes interpreted as making them better or keeping them safe. However, this may conflict with service users' perceptions, who, like other people, accept that risk is part of life.

Beneficence

Professionals' prioritisation of a beneficent, caring approach may be reinforced by concern for their own professional standing should something go wrong when they facilitate risk-taking. It can be difficult to construe 'duty of care' as incorporating duty to hear and act upon service users' opinions, if professionals see problems ahead.

Protection from abuse

If a person with dementia is at risk of abuse (see Chapter 59), the obvious solution (guided by the principle of non-maleficence) is to remove the vulnerable person from the potential abuser or vice versa. However, the person with dementia may feel that the relationship is more important than avoiding risk. In this case, a negotiated support programme to minimise stress and monitor the situation can be a fairer and more acceptable solution.

Informed consent

All health and social care interventions (e.g. taking medicine, being helped to wash) are dependent on service users' understanding and agreement. However, for people with dementia, understanding can be difficult to achieve if their mental capacity is weakened and they do not comprehend the options. In this situation, the autonomy of the person should be promoted by aiding decision-making (e.g. by using simple language, pictures or metaphors), and if this is unsuccessful, by considering the person's previous attitudes (as described by friends or family) and combining this information with other considerations so as to make a decision (guided by beneficence) in the person's best interest (see Chapter 62).

Truth telling and 'therapeutic lies'

In the later stages of dementia, people may be disorientated in time, person and place. They may believe, for example, that their parents are alive when they are not and ask for them continuously. Although professionals (and family carers) believe in honesty, they may feel that a lie is less harmful than repeatedly breaking distressing news (Chapter 50).

Justice and considering others

The needs of people with dementia often lead to them being cared for by family members at home; sometimes this falls upon one person, whose life becomes gradually more constrained. The pressure on the caregiver can be significantly stressful and ill health can be a result. In valuing people with dementia, it is also an ethical priority, driven by the principle of justice, to value and support those who provide care.

61 Advocacy

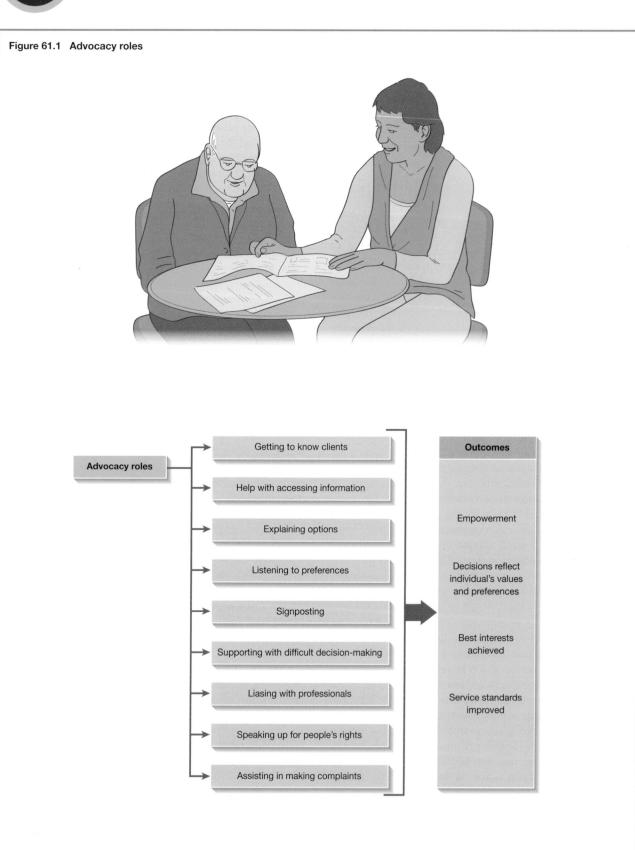

Figure 61.1   Advocacy roles

Advocacy roles
- Getting to know clients
- Help with accessing information
- Explaining options
- Listening to preferences
- Signposting
- Supporting with difficult decision-making
- Liasing with professionals
- Speaking up for people's rights
- Assisting in making complaints

Outcomes

Empowerment

Decisions reflect individual's values and preferences

Best interests achieved

Service standards improved

Dementia Care at a Glance, First Edition. Catharine Jenkins, Laura Ginesi and Bernie Keenan. © 2016 by John Wiley & Sons, Ltd. Published 2016 by John Wiley & Sons, Ltd.
Companion website: www.ataglanceseries.com/nursing/dementiacare

Speaking up for another person's interests

Advocacy is the process of expressing the views and standing up for the interests of a person who is not able to do so independently. It can involve safeguarding their rights, arguing their corner and contributing to decision-making from a perspective of understanding the person's wishes (Figure 61.1). People with dementia and other mental health problems or learning disabilities may not be able to understand complex issues that lie behind a difficult decision or its consequences. They may not be able to argue or express their thoughts and feelings coherently. There is a risk that decisions are taken on their behalf, made in the interests of organisations or other individuals, rather than the service user themselves. A diagnosis of dementia can sometimes mean that a person's views are not taken seriously, so sometimes complaints are ignored. Sometimes staff or family members do not have the skills, inclination or time to assist people to come to their own decision. People with dementia are adults and citizens with the right to be heard, and assisted if necessary, to make autonomous decisions about their own lives. Occasionally abusive situations arise and the skills of an advocate are required to protect a person with dementia.

Being an advocate for a person with dementia can be a challenging role and may conflict with other aspects of a professional's activities (or relationships in the case of family or friend advocates). Although nurses, social workers and other health and social care workers see being an advocate for service users' interests as part of their job description (and included in professional Codes of Conduct), they are not always in a position to truly take the side of the individual. For example, a person with dementia may indicate a wish to carry out a risky activity and the nurse may want to protect them, or a junior staff member may be in a less powerful position than a consultant and struggle to be heard within the multi-disciplinary team. Therefore, there is also a need for independent trained advocates.

Skills of advocates

Advocates must be able to quickly form a rapport with the person with dementia and have excellent listening skills in order to understand their perceptions, feelings and wishes. They need to be able to frame questions so that the person with dementia understands them, and also explain potential outcomes in a way that enables retention for someone with poor short-term memory. Advocates must believe in the rights of people with dementia and the importance of maximising their autonomy. This may mean learning about the person's life history and previous decisions, accessing records, finding and approaching family members and investigating whether a person has appointed someone to have lasting power of attorney (LPA). If so, they would liaise and devolve the decision-making to this person, unless they had concerns about whether the LPA was acting in the person's best interests. If the advocate concludes (by using the two-step test of the Mental Capacity Act (2005); Chapter 62) that the person with dementia does not have capacity to contribute towards making a specific decision and has no one else who can help them, they then contribute to making decisions on the person's behalf. They use understanding of the person and the situation's potential outcomes to guide them in working in the individual's best

interests. The advocate needs to be able to explain their working process and its outcome to the multi-disciplinary team, some of whom may feel the involvement of an 'outsider' is unnecessary. Therefore, the advocate needs to be focused articulate and brave. The advocate also needs to be able to gather information quickly, liaise respectfully and assertively with others and write clear concise reports quickly. If their report is ignored or overlooked they need to be prepared to re-challenge the lead decision-maker.

External agencies

Generally a family member or friend who knows them well and is motivated to stand up for their interests supports a person with dementia. However, there are some people with dementia who are isolated and do not have a suitable informal advocate. In this situation, multi-disciplinary team members can find via Patient Advice and Liaison Services (PALS) in hospital environments, or Citizens' Advice, Age UK or other organisations in the local community (see Chapter 13). (Worldadvocacy.com provides links to advocacy organisations internationally.)

Independent mental capacity advocates

Important decisions such as a move to new accommodation or relating to medical treatment can sometimes be a cause for conflict. Family members may not agree or there may be suggestions that decisions are not being made in the best interests of the person with dementia. Independent Mental Capacity Advocates (IMCAs) were established through the Mental Capacity Act (2005) (and similar legislation elsewhere, e.g. The Adults with Incapacity (Scotland) Act 2000) to support the autonomy of people who may lack capacity (Chapter 62). If the person with dementia has not appointed an LPA, then the IMCA takes the lead in establishing what the person's 'best interests' are and ensuring they are upheld. IMCAs are usually employees of existing advocacy agencies, with additional specialised training.

Collective advocacy

People with dementia as advocates

People with dementia as a group have the right to have their voices heard. Increasingly they are creating and developing opportunities to speak out about their needs and rights. People with dementia who speak at conferences, write for newsletters and journals and contribute to training are advocating for the well-being of the group to which they belong.

Third sector organisations

The Alzheimer's Society and other organisations internationally advocate for people with dementia as a group. These organisations collaborate to influence and direct government and local policy so that the rights of people with dementia are upheld. They offer a forum within which people with dementia can feel safe in expressing their opinions and contributing to national debates. They have been successful in raising public awareness and guiding attitudes so as to reduce stigma and promote inclusion and are involved in ongoing campaigns about the structure and financing of health and social care.

62 Mental capacity

Figure 62.1 Mental capacity

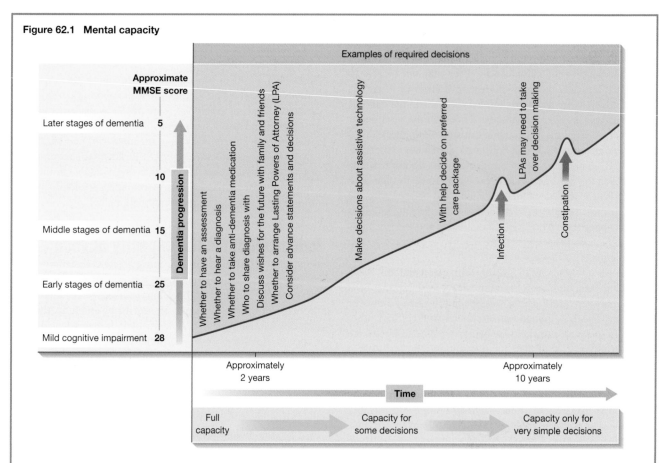

Figure 62.2 Principles of the UK Mental Capacity Act (2005)

A person:

- Must be assumed to have capacity – a diagnosis, age or appearance should not lead to assumptions about lack of capacity
- Has the right to be helped to make decisions
- Has the right to make 'unwise' decisions

...and if the person is not able to make a decision:

- It should be made in his or her best interests
- And should be made so that the outcome is least restrictive

Figure 62.3 Deprivation of Liberty Safeguards (DoLS) which apply in England and Wales

If a person over 18, with dementia (or another mental disorder or disability) lacks capacity to make health-related decisions for themselves, and is in hospital or a care home, they may be protected by DoLS legislation

DoLS allow staff to act in the best interest of a person who lacks capacity to make relevant decisions by:

- Restricting their liberty, for example, distracting a person who wishes to leave a care home, but who would be unsafe on the roads or get lost
- Restraining a person who needs a bath following an episode of incontinence, but who does not understand this and resists help

Authorisation to use DoLS legislation needs to be obtained from the Local Authority or Primary Care Trust. A representative, (a friend or family member) is appointed to ensure care is provided in the least restrictive way. If the person wishes to challenge a DoLS authorisation, they can apply to the Court of Protection. They have the right to an Independent Mental Capacity Advocate (IMCA)

Dementia Care at a Glance, First Edition. Catharine Jenkins, Laura Ginesi and Bernie Keenan. © 2016 by John Wiley & Sons, Ltd. Published 2016 by John Wiley & Sons, Ltd.
Companion website: www.ataglanceseries.com/nursing/dementiacare

Defining capacity

Mental capacity refers to the ability to make decisions. It is relevant to the lives of people with dementia because the gradual deterioration associated with dementia affects a person's ability to understand information and to weigh it up and then come to a decision. However, the nature of a person's ability to make a decision is not determined by the diagnosis. Each person is unique, the types of dementia affect people differently, and the journey through the stages is individual. In addition, some decisions are easier than others (e.g. which cardigan to wear as opposed to how to manage investments) and again that depends not only on the decision itself but also on the person's level of education, communication abilities and personal history and experiences. Therefore, a person cannot be said to lack capacity just because they have a diagnosis of dementia (or any other condition) or because they are up against a decision they find impossible to make. A person-centred approach that respects autonomy involves assuming that the person does have capacity, and then if it seems that a particular decision is difficult to make, the person should be assisted to make his or her own decision.

Fluctuating abilities

People with dementia often experience fluctuation in their orientation, cognition and communication abilities. For example, most people are brighter in the morning and then become more tired and sometimes more disorientated in the late afternoon and evening (Chapter 55). Physical causes can disrupt mental well-being, so infection, constipation or pain can affect concentration and understanding (Chapters 21 and 28). If there is an important decision to be made, it is sensible to wait until the person is at their best so that they can make their own decision.

The progression of dementia: decision-making needs

Most people make major decisions in consultation with people they trust. For most people, there is a sliding scale in which they make some decisions independently and others with help. Similarly, people with dementia are able to make some decisions themselves, but need help with more complex issues. As their dementia progresses, the person may gradually need more help, with less complicated decisions (Figure 62.1). Eventually he or she may not be able to make their own decisions and need a substitute decision-maker who will protect their interests.

The Mental Capacity Act (2005)

The purpose of this legislation (which applies in England and Wales) is to empower people who may have weakened capacity and to protect them so that any decisions that other people make on their behalf are made in their best interests (Figure 62.2). Similar legislation exists elsewhere (e.g. The Adults with Incapacity (Scotland) Act 2000 and in the United States, Canada and Australia). Capacity is considered to be 'decision-specific' (rather than 'on/off') and in the United Kingdom, a two-step test is used to decide whether someone has capacity for that decision.

Step 1: Has the person got a disorder of their mind or brain?
Step 2: If so, in relation to the decision, can the person

- Understand the issues related to the decision
- Retain the information long enough to …
- Weigh it up
- And then communicate their decision (by any means)

If the person with dementia does not have capacity for that decision, then relevant people will make the decision in their best interest.

Planning ahead

Any person can make plans for the future, anticipating that they may lose capacity for important decisions. The options are:

- An advance care plan involving 'advance statements' about preferred care. This is not legally binding but is helpful to family and professionals aiming to care for someone as they would wish.
- Advance decisions (sometimes referred to as a 'living will' and also previously known as 'advance directives') are legally binding and should be written, witnessed and signed. These involve *refusal* of certain treatments, even if they are life-saving (though cannot be used to refuse food and drink on behalf of their future self, nor plan for assisted suicide in the United Kingdom).
- It is also possible to arrange for proxy (stand-in) decision makers who would be willing to act in the person's interests on their behalf if need be. These are called 'lasting powers of attorney' (LPA), and in the United Kingdom, law can be appointed to deal with Health and Welfare or Finances, or both (see Direct.Gov website).

Assistance with decision-making

People with dementia may require assistance to make decisions. The person helping has the role of making the factors clearer rather than guiding the person in their decision. To do this, they can:

- Choose a time when the person is most lucid
- Keep background noise to a minimum and make sure the person can see clearly
- Explain the context in simple language, then outline the decision
- Use familiar terminology. Pictures can sometimes help
- Break down the problem into small chunks
- Listen carefully to the person's replies, read their non-verbal communication and respond sensitively
- Build up to the decision in simple steps, checking for understanding (not yes/no, but by using their own words)
- Summarise and check back with the person to confirm the decision
- Aim to ascertain the person's general beliefs so as to be able to check that the conclusion 'fits' and is accurately understood
- Make notes on the conversation and date them. The person with dementia may also wish to sign the record

Best interests

If the person is unable to make their own decision, then a decision must be made for them in their best interest. If someone has an LPA, the LPA would decide. Otherwise, the multi-disciplinary team (for a health or social care matter) or solicitor (for legal matters) would lead. If the person has recorded their wishes, these should be followed, and anything relevant they have said or done in the past should be taken into account. Independent Mental Capacity Advocates can also be used if a situation is contested. Under the Mental Capacity Act (2005), people with dementia may also take part in research, even if it is not directly in their own interests, if it is aiming to improve the treatment or care of people with the same condition and taking part is in line with the person's known belief system.

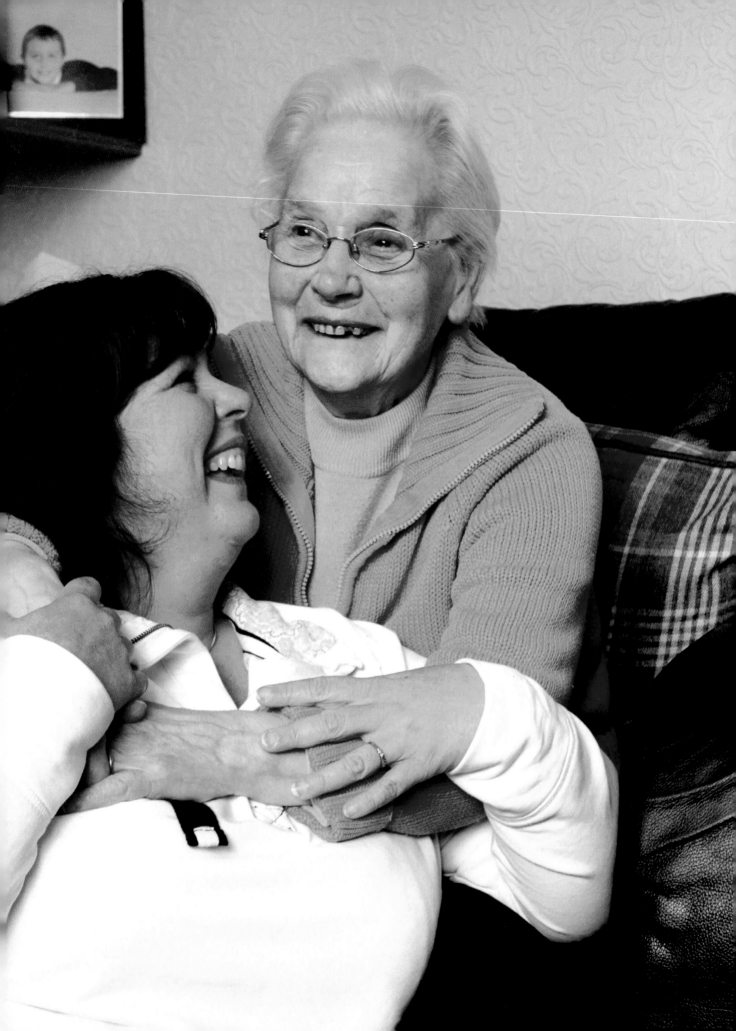

The future

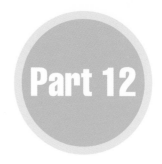

Part 12

63 Leadership issues

Figure 63.1   Leadership qualities for dementia care

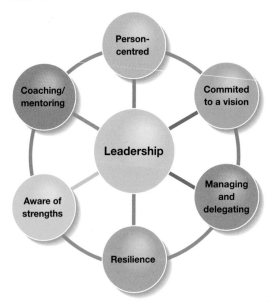

Table 63.1   The impact of good leadership on dementia care, for example, in a care home

On multi-disciplinary teams	On people with dementia and families
A clear vision of high-quality care and expectation that this will be offered at all times	They can relax knowing high quality care is the norm
Clarity about roles and responsibilities	They will be signposted to the appropriate team member according to expressed need
Team members know they can approach the leader if they have a problem	Needs are met more quickly and cheerfully – it does not feel as if asking is 'a bother'
Staff help each other and are happy to carry out tasks outside their role description	Any difficulties can be resolved before they escalate
A problem-solving culture	Any difficulties are viewed as manageable and strategies are designed and tested to resolve them
Colleagues feel valued by the leader	Team members follow the 'model' of valuing and demonstrate similar feelings and behaviours while valuing those they look after
Colleagues appreciate each other's skills and qualities	Team members learn from each other so that care quality is always improving
Confidence – staff are happy to explain their work and welcome visitors	Able to visit the unit freely and look forward to spending time in each other's company
Team members look out for each other and are mutually supportive	Life is more spontaneous, flexible and responsive to personal preferences
Enhanced creativity – staff feel empowered to try out new ideas	A warm, safe and supportive atmosphere is maintained
Reduced absence from work and reduced turnover of staff	People with dementia get to know their carers well and feel safe with them. Staff members get to know the personalities and histories of the people they look after and feel genuinely attached to them

Dementia Care at a Glance, First Edition. Catharine Jenkins, Laura Ginesi and Bernie Keenan. © 2016 by John Wiley & Sons, Ltd. Published 2016 by John Wiley & Sons, Ltd.
Companion website: www.ataglanceseries.com/nursing/dementiacare

eople with dementia need sensitive, positive, patient, emotionally responsive and committed carers. They need long-term emotional connections with people who know them and care about them. The relationships between care providers and those they look after is essential to service-users' well-being, but because roles can be stressful staff need support, mentoring and coaching to enable them to enhance the care they offer and to carry on giving of their best. Meeting the emotional and practical needs of care workers is therefore as important as meeting those of service-users and good leadership is key to achieving this (Figure 63.1).

Person-centred leadership for care

Leadership is the behaviour that makes other people want to follow. It involves having a strong vision of what the person or organisation is aiming for and communicating this to others in a way that engages and makes them feel emotionally and practically committed to being part of making it happen. Leadership roles often involve some management responsibilities, for example, in recruitment, delegating tasks, organising finances and writing policies, but these are tools of leadership rather than the end results. It is important that the management aspects of organisational behaviour are congruent with its stated (person-centred) aims so that team members can feel that the ideals are genuinely held and worth their commitment.

Purpose and motivation

Leaders of health and social care teams need to have a vision of what they are aiming for, both for current day-to-day practice and for future developments. The vision – for example, 'we will provide care that enables each person with dementia to live an enjoyable, meaningful life where they feel they are a valuable individual in a caring community' – then drives the leader's behaviour, as all their actions communicate commitment to this vision. As people with dementia need a sense of purpose, so too do those involved in all levels of care. Working with a sense of purpose promotes job satisfaction, which then reinforces commitment.

Person-centred leadership qualities

People in leadership roles need to promote this commitment within their sphere of influence, in a way that brings their colleagues on board so that everyone works together, feeling they are part of something that is bigger than them and that is significant and rewarding (Table 63.1). The qualities needed to motivate and facilitate change are similar to those required for person-centred dementia care. Leaders need to respond sensitively to those they lead, considering individual's identities and how their support and encouragement can build the worker's identity further within the role. A strong sense of identity is mutually reinforced, so the leader has the opportunity to recognise strengths and also to work with the person on any areas that need to be addressed. They may also learn from those they lead. While leaders need to be brave in acknowledging their own emotions and those of others, they do not aim to confront people or control them but rather to engage with them in a person-centred way so that the worker is drawn along rather than feeling resistant to change.

The leader achieves this through the use of approaches such as:

- Listening
- Encouraging
- Guiding
- Supporting
- Modelling
- Challenging (but in a manner that avoids loss of face)
- Delegating leadership opportunities
- Communicating through words and actions
- Thanking

Relationship-centred care: needs of staff

Leaders consider the emotional needs of their colleagues, much as they consider the needs of service users, because person-centred care needs to come from a person-centred way of being, which is then reflected in everything a person does and says. Working in the field of dementia care is immensely rewarding but can also be hard work. The challenges of providing care to people with dementia can mean that workers are at risk of physical and emotional exhaustion. Services may be under-resourced and the people who deliver hands-on care tend to be paid low wages. The rewards of the work are not financial but come through job satisfaction and a sense that they have made a positive difference to another's life (Table 63.1).

Transformational leadership

Transformational leaders achieve change in organisations by serving the vision that they believe in and those they lead. They take a 'hearts and minds' approach to influencing both carers and colleagues and empower others to commit to action towards the shared goal and take on leadership characteristics for themselves. Transformational leaders perceive their role as a mission; their beliefs and values are central to who they are. Their genuine enthusiasm and dedication drive their own behaviour and motivates others.

Collaborative leadership

In large complex organisations, one leader may not be able to change a care culture. 'Collaborative leadership' involves people at all levels committing to positively influencing the organisational culture within the parameters of their roles.

Changing care cultures

Person-centredness refers to an approach to dementia care that puts the person's experience at the centre: everything done for and with that individual should be aimed towards making him or her feel emotionally connected with others and valuable. In the past, dementia care was very task-oriented and care was arranged around the timetable of the organisation or the priorities of care providers. Even though Kitwood's work (1997) (Chapter 15) and the approach he promoted are well known, care environments still often reflect the old culture. It is not easy to influence ingrained habits that are based on entrenched norms and values. People who want to take a lead in providing genuine person-centred care for those who are affected by dementia need to be courageous in arguing for change and 'leading upwards'. Confidence drawn from the belief that change is essential and achievable motivates leaders at all levels. Everything done today helps construct the future that we want and every interaction has meaning and influences others. Person-centred leadership is congruent with valuing people with dementia, ones' colleagues and oneself.

64 Research

Figure 64.1 The methodological frameworks for health-related research

Quantitative research	Qualitative research
☐ Discovering facts about phenomena	☐ Understanding human behaviour is a key concern
☐ Assumes measureable reality	☐ Assumes a dynamic reality
☐ Data collected through measurement	☐ Data collected through participant observation, questionnaires, interviews, etc.
☐ Data analysed and reported in terms of numerical comparisons and statistical inferences	☐ Data analysed by thematic frameworks based on participants descriptions and responses

Figure 64.2 Possible targets for research in dementia

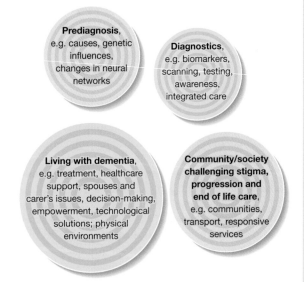

Prediagnosis, e.g. causes, genetic influences, changes in neural networks

Diagnostics, e.g. biomarkers, scanning, testing, awareness, integrated care

Living with dementia, e.g. treatment, healthcare support, spouses and carer's issues, decision-making, empowerment, technological solutions; physical environments

Community/society challenging stigma, progression and end of life care, e.g. communities, transport, responsive services

Figure 64.3 Some outcome markers used in research into dementia

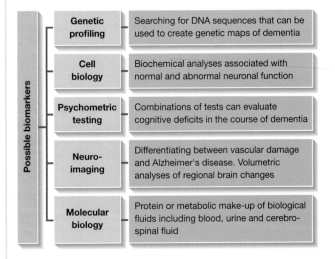

Possible biomarkers

Genetic profiling	Searching for DNA sequences that can be used to create genetic maps of dementia
Cell biology	Biochemical analyses associated with normal and abnormal neuronal function
Psychometric testing	Combinations of tests can evaluate cognitive deficits in the course of dementia
Neuro-imaging	Differentiating between vascular damage and Alzheimer's disease. Volumetric analyses of regional brain changes
Molecular biology	Protein or metabolic make-up of biological fluids including blood, urine and cerebro-spinal fluid

Figure 64.5 Relative funding of research into major diseases (UK; 2007/2008)

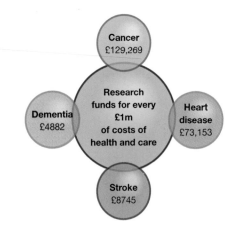

Cancer £129,269

Research funds for every £1m of costs of health and care

Dementia £4882

Heart disease £73,153

Stroke £8745

Figure 64.4 The discovery and development of new treatments and medications can take many years as each new phase of the research builds on knowledge gained from previous ones. Clinical trials follow strict pre-defined protocols to ensure safety and validity of results

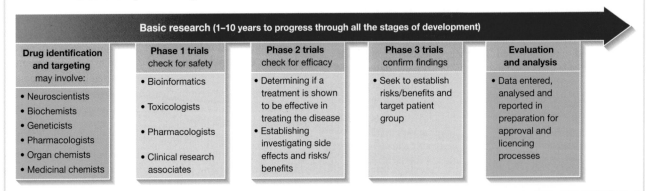

Basic research (1–10 years to progress through all the stages of development)

Drug identification and targeting may involve:	Phase 1 trials check for safety	Phase 2 trials check for efficacy	Phase 3 trials confirm findings	Evaluation and analysis
• Neuroscientists • Biochemists • Geneticists • Pharmacologists • Organ chemists • Medicinal chemists	• Bioinformatics • Toxicologists • Pharmacologists • Clinical research associates	• Determining if a treatment is shown to be effective in treating the disease • Establishing investigating side effects and risks/benefits	• Seek to establish risks/benefits and target patient group	• Data entered, analysed and reported in preparation for approval and licencing processes

Dementia Care at a Glance, First Edition. Catharine Jenkins, Laura Ginesi and Bernie Keenan. © 2016 by John Wiley & Sons, Ltd. Published 2016 by John Wiley & Sons, Ltd.
Companion website: www.ataglanceseries.com/nursing/dementiacare

In general, research offers hope for successful treatment and better management of dementia in the future and improved quality of life for people with dementia and their loved ones. However, researching dementia is challenging because those who are affected often have very complex health needs because they are living with additional medical condition(s) or disability.

Advances in dementia care arise from innovative ideas and approaches that have been developed through research investigations in which people investigate health in a systematic way in order to answer a question (see Figure 64.1). Attention is turning towards better understanding of the changes that are typical of many neurodegenerative disorders – sporadic and inherited – including Alzheimer's disease.

Basic research into dementia

Investigations in laboratories generally point the way to new methods that offer possibility for improved outcomes for people with dementia (Figure 64.2). An important focus is better understanding of the earliest stages of cognitive problems through understanding the types of genetic changes (mutations) that increase risk.

Dementia and lost memories are the result of dying neurons, so drugs in development take aim at a variety of neural mechanisms, for example, abnormalities in the microtubule-associated protein called tau or build-up of amyloid fragments (see Chapters 5, 6 and 7). Such changes can build up 10–15 years before clinical symptoms like memory loss appear, so biomarkers (Figure 64.3) could be vital tools that have potential for:

- Better diagnostic techniques
- Earlier detection of disease and progression
- Potential target for novel drug therapies
- Better management of predictors of pathology, e.g. concussion or stroke, with the aim of reducing dementia in the longer term.

The advantage of laboratory-based investigations is that they take place under controlled conditions, allowing neuroscientists to manipulate variables, for example, different drug treatments and to measure outcomes of the experiment. The aim of much of this basic research is to curb the onset of the disease before the worst symptoms manifest themselves, but, to date, none of the approaches are proved to be able to stop dementia in its tracks and offer tangible opportunities for protecting neurons and slowing the course of the disease.

Qualitative research

Qualitative research is designed to study the impact and effects of the disease on the individual such as quality of life, costs, care and comfort (Figure 64.1). Meaningful research findings can help to support wider, more open debate related to the funding of high-quality health and social care that meets the needs of people affected by dementia who may feel lonely, isolated and stigmatised by their communities. However, this raises a need for consideration of the extent to which the circumstances and context of research interventions have an impact in the real world of service provision.

Clinical trials

A disadvantage of basic research is difficulty in predicting how a new treatment/medication/intervention may act in any one individual. Randomised controlled trials (see Figure 64.5) test the efficacy of new medications, agents or factors that impact on cognitive function, skills, thinking or behaviour, which may have promise in treating or preventing dementia.

A major challenge for researchers is that people with dementia may suffer from several different chronic conditions; medications taken in combination can lead to a situation called polypharmacy (Chapter 33) in which the actions of drugs and the way the body handles them are altered. This means that people who have dementia are prone to adverse reactions, so new treatments always carry risks as well as potential benefits. Clinical studies must be very carefully and ethically designed to protect vulnerable people from unnecessary adverse effects (see Figure 64.4). Unfortunately, some trials have had to be stopped early due to unforeseen side effects. Trials are costly and the lack of success has led pharmaceutical companies to become more cautious about further investment in similar trials.

Funding for research into dementia

Limited funding has meant that there have been few research breakthroughs or advances in treatment for dementia. In the United Kingdom alone, dementia currently costs an estimated £23 billion per year, which is more than the combined costs of cancer, stroke and heart disease. However, the distribution of research funding is biased in favour of cancer and coronary heart disease rather than neurological disorders (see Figure 64.5).

Collaborative research groups bring together people who have overlapping, active interests, but different expertise and perspectives on a research problem. It is essential that people with dementia and their caregivers be included in research, as they have 'lived experience' of the condition and have much to contribute.

Researching well-being, quality of life and training

Although many who are living with dementia say they are living well, the behavioural and psychological symptoms of dementia can be distressing for the person with dementia themselves and contribute to carer stress. Since the numbers of people with dementia and informal caregivers are growing worldwide, there is an urgent need to explore the impact of alternative methods of healthcare system practices and carer support. There are many uncertainties related to dementia that can be addressed by involving people who have dementia, their families and other carers in setting the research agenda.

Examples of current research

- Antibodies that block the process of synapse disintegration in Alzheimer's disease have been identified, raising hopes for a treatment to combat early cognitive decline in the disease.
- High doses of the antibiotic minocycline are being tested to see whether they reduce inflammation in the brain.
- Non-pharmacological interventions provided by caregivers may reduce the frequency and severity of symptoms and can reduce caregiver burden, with effect sizes similar to those associated with medications, but the evidence base needs to be improved.
- Approaches to training professional carers of people with dementia, for example, doctors and nurses, are being evaluated with a view to exploring which methods help professionals embed person-centred approaches in their practice, innovate and lead on changing cultures of care.

65 Conclusion

Figure 65.1 The future of dementia

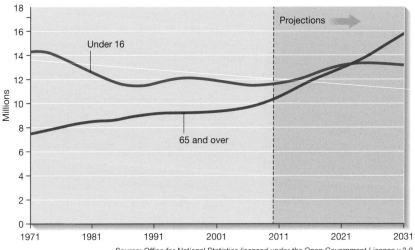

The Office of National Statistics has estimated that compared to 2011 in 2021 there will be 24% more people aged 65+ and 39% more people aged 85+ in England.

In 2030, (compared to 2010) there will be 51% more people aged 65+ and 101% more people aged 85+

Source: *Office for National Statistics licensed under the Open Government Licence v.3.0*

Figure 65.2 Future projections

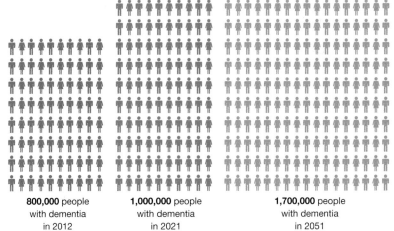

The number of people in the UK with dementia will double in the next 40 years

👤 = 10,000 people

800,000 people with dementia in 2012

1,000,000 people with dementia in 2021

1,700,000 people with dementia in 2051

Source: *Reproduced with permission of the Alzheimer's Society*

Table 65.1 The context of a rapidly developing speciality

- The demographics of an ageing population

- The relationship between unhealthy lifestyles and dementia

- Possibilities for earlier diagnosis, resulting in higher numbers of people in early stages of dementia who are able to articulate their expectations

- Challenges to ageist assumptions related to older peoples' needs and use of resources

- The context of budget restrictions and escalating care costs

- Alignment of national and international pressure groups (e.g. Alzheimers International and the Alzheimer's Society (UK)) with politicians, giving stronger voice and representation to people with dementia and giving them input to driving policy and legislation

- Lack of a medical breakthrough for either prevention or cure, despite millions of pounds worth of research

- Scandals related to abusive care in hospitals and care homes

- The changing nature of patients in general hospitals – more will be older, more will have very complex needs and many, or in some wards, most, will have dementia

- High-profile media campaigns highlighting both alarmist '1 in 3' and reassuring 'it is possible to live well with dementia' messages

- Increasing awareness that in the context of limited resources and the preferences of most people with dementia to live at home, local communities will have to develop the capacity to offer much more informal support

Dementia Care at a Glance, First Edition. Catharine Jenkins, Laura Ginesi and Bernie Keenan. © 2016 by John Wiley & Sons, Ltd. Published 2016 by John Wiley & Sons, Ltd.
Companion website: www.ataglanceseries.com/nursing/dementiacare

Perceptions of the field of dementia care have changed dramatically in recent years. When Kitwood wrote *Dementia Reconsidered: The Person Comes First* in 1997 (Chapter 15), dementia care was organised around a medical model in which any treatment only aimed to control behaviour. Long stigmatised (in the Western world) by an ageist society that valued intellectual functioning and usefulness above other human qualities, dementia care was considered a professional backwater within which therapeutic nihilism ruled.

Understandings of dementia

The number of people with dementia is now growing exponentially on a global scale, reflecting worldwide demographic patterns in which larger numbers are surviving into old age and experiencing associated long-term conditions, including dementia (Figure 65.1). Southern and Eastern worldviews (see Chapter 16) have a lot to teach about including people with dementia and valuing their lives holistically, including the insight that can be gained from listening to people with dementia. The common perception in traditional societies and by lay people worldwide of dementia as a natural part of ageing can be seen as protective of a person's social standing and less stigmatising than a westernised 'disease' perception. While some professionals share the opinion that dementia is 'part of normal ageing', for the most part the role of degenerative processes in the brain is acknowledged and the experience of dementia is constructed as a bio-psycho-social phenomenon in which physiological changes combine with a person's emotions, relationships and situations in society.

Person-centredness

The challenge in Kitwood's work to 'see the person' began the revolution towards 'person-centred' care, which valued the experience of the person with dementia and considered a more holistic view of the person. Based on a humanistic model, the central message of hope – that it is possible to maintain the well-being of those with dementia through relationships and interventions that support 'personhood' or identity – offered an opportunity for health and social care professionals to offer positive alternatives based on qualities and skills rather than prescriptions and controlling regimes.

In the family context, though, person-centred care often fell on the shoulders of one person (usually a wife or daughter), while in care homes care it has usually been provided by female under-trained, under-paid and under-valued care workers, who in common with family carers, were often expected to put their own needs on hold in favour of those they look after. Lack of 'success' in achieving well-being for cared-for people in these circumstances has been construed as neglect by individuals rather than a consequence of a combination of factors including lack of guidance, under-resourcing and exploitation deriving from stigmatising values.

Relationship-centred care

Under-recognition of caring roles was challenged by Nolan's (2006) concept of relationship-centred care which raised awareness of the needs of all parties (the person with dementia, family carers and professional carers) for senses of security, belonging, purpose, continuity, significance and fulfilment/achievement. Recent information (Alzheimer's Society, 2014a) has revealed that many people with dementia feel lonely, even within their own communities, so it seems many of these needs are still not being met.

A social model in practice

Recent initiatives in the United Kingdom, 'Dementia Friends' and 'Dementia Friendly Communities', have emphasised social inclusion and the potential for everyone to commit to taking part in promoting the well-being of members of the community with dementia. Within a social model of understanding, dementia is reframed as a disability for which others should make reasonable adjustments and the dementia friends initiatives highlight the important roles of the public both at home and at work in business and service industries in attaining wider acceptance and support of those with dementia.

Modern cohorts of older people

New generations of people, diagnosed much earlier in the course of the condition, well educated, confident, computer literate and well informed, are currently challenging professionals and putting their own mark on the field. They are raising public awareness of the myths and stigma and contributing to the education of health and social care professionals. In expecting professional, personally tailored, high-quality care that recognises and responds to individual needs, they are setting the bar so that the rhetoric of 'person-centred' care is matched by reality in which the care actually revolves around the person – who they are – what they need and how they would like it to be provided.

Contentious issues

Standards of care

Highest standards of care are not universal. In hospitals, care homes and the community, the approach to care is sometimes driven by financial priorities rather than service users' quality of life. People with dementia may find that their personal care is rushed, that no one listens to them and that they are treated more like parcels than people. Social environments where this approach is acceptable may provide the conditions in which neglect and abuse can develop. Poor standards of care should be challenged.

End-of-life debates

The autonomy of people with dementia is protected by legislation in most countries. People with the capacity to make decisions have power over their future selves, to the extent that they can refuse treatment on their future self's behalf and in some countries decide upon assisted suicide in advance of deterioration of their condition. The choice to refuse life as a person in the later stages of dementia divides those who would celebrate the opportunity to avoid suffering from those who believe life with dementia has equal human value. Discriminatory perceptions of people with dementia as 'burdens', could lead to pressure being put on them to request assistance to die for the sake of other people rather than themselves.

Research: cure, care or prevention?

Despite huge investments, there is still a lack of viable anti-dementia drugs on the near horizon. It is becoming increasingly clear that any treatments will have to be given some time before symptoms emerge and their success will be dependent on biomarker identifiers. Less well-funded research into care has investigated alternative models (e.g. The Enriched Care Model), the process of culture change, competency frameworks to identify the attitudes, knowledge and skills required by different professionals and how to educate and empower health and social care professionals so that they are able to promote and embed person-centred approaches within their organisations.

Recent research into the causes of dementia and its prevention seems to be indicating a higher than expected lifestyle component, where obesity, alcohol use and lack of exercise play a part in its development. Future stigmatising stereotypes could give rise to a blame culture in which people with dementia are considered responsible for their own misfortune, while concerns about costs and funding of care could alienate younger generations.

Funding and achieving high-quality care

'Living well with dementia' requires adjustments to the physical environment, the social environment and the level of respect accorded to those responsible for making the slogan a reality. Family carers and paid carers carry out roles that can be hard physical work, emotionally testing and demand high levels of patience and specialised communication skills. Yet this work is still perceived to be low status, and workers receive low pay. Most are women; many have English as a second language and minimal education, but have cultural values which promote respectful attitudes to older people. In many situations, the vulnerable are being cared for by the exploited.

Learning for the future

The field of dementia care is in a state of flux, reflecting both serious concerns about financial costs and the difficulties of promoting acceptable standards of care and feelings of optimism related to the positive potential of the voices of people with dementia being heard within their communities, in education and training and in contributing to policymaking and legislation.

Many countries now have dementia strategies and have made commitments to invest in research, standards of care and health promotion campaigns. Awareness-raising programmes mean that more people recognise the symptoms associated with dementia and know to seek support. Concerns arising from investigations into failures in standards of care and media campaigns resulted in measures to monitor care standards and introduce dementia care education throughout the workforce. Professionalisation of care workers together with greater visibility of people with dementia challenging stigma, contributing to health and social care staff training and demanding access to a choice of flexible services within local communities, should raise the profile of the speciality further.

Despite the history of old cultures of dementia care, there is cause for hope. Current factors that support optimism include:

- Greater understanding of causative factors and how promoting lifetime well-being is an investment for old age
- Improved knowledge of dementia-related processes in the brain, which ultimately should underpin development of preventative therapies
- Greater understanding of what good-quality care looks like and how and where it should be provided
- More insight into how to educate a committed, effective dementia care workforce who are recognised for their skills and expertise
- Government commitments to older cohorts of voters
- Open discussion of funding alternatives for high-quality care

In valuing people with dementia, it is important to value those who support them. The various issues covered in this book indicate the complex mix of physical, emotional, attitudinal, therapeutic and social interventions which make a difference to the lives of people with dementia.

We hope that the information presented in this book will inspire and assist all those involved in the field of dementia care to develop deeper understanding of the potential they have to make a difference and to promote the well-being of people living with dementia now and in the future.

References

Alzheimer's Society. (2012). Dementia 2012: a national challenge. Available at: http://www.alzheimers.org.uk/dementia2012 (accessed on 14 November 2014).

Alzheimer's Society. (2014a). Dementia 2014: opportunity for change. Available at: http://www.alzheimers.org.uk/site/scripts/download_info.php?fileID=2317 (accessed on 14 November 2014).

Alzheimer's Society. (2014b). Singing for the brain. Available at: http://www.alzheimers.org.uk/site/scripts/documents_info.php?documentID=760 (accessed on 14 November 2014).

BAPEN. (2013). Malnutrition universal screening tool. Available at: http://www.bapen.org.uk/screening-for-malnutrition/must/introducing-must (accessed on 14 November 2014).

Block SM. (2009). *The Story of Forgetting*. London: Faber & Faber.

Brooker D. (2007). *Person Centred Dementia Care: Making Services Better*. London: Jessica Kingsley Publishers.

Bryden C. (2005). *Dancing with Dementia: My Story of Living Positively with Dementia*. London: Jessica Kingsley Publishers.

Bute J. (2014). Glorious opportunity. Available at: http://www.gloriousopportunity.org/ (accessed on 14 November 2014).

Mental Capacity ActEuropean Pressure Ulcer Advisory Panel; National Pressure Ulcer Advisory Panel. (2009). Treatment of pressure ulcers: quick reference guide. Available at: http://www.epuap.org/guidelines/Final_Quick_Treatment.pdf (accessed on 3 November 2014).

Feil N. (1993). *The Validation Breakthrough: Simple Techniques for Communicating with People with Alzheimer's Type Dementia*. Baltimore: Health Professions Press.

Genova L. (2009). *Still Alice: A Novel*. New York: Gallery Books.

Human Rights Act. (1998). Available at: http://www.legislation.gov.uk/ukpga/1998/42/contents (accessed on 14 November 2014).

Inouye SK, van Dyck CH, Alessi CA, Balkin S, Siegal AP, Horwitz RI. (1990). Clarifying confusion: the confusion assessment method. A new method for detection of delirium. *Annals of Internal Medicine*, 113, 941–948. The confusion assessment method (CAM) diagnostic algorithm. Available at: http://www.guysandstthomas.nhs.uk/resources/our-services/acute-medicine-gi-surgery/elderly-care/cam-diagnostic-algorithm.pdf (accessed on 14 November 2014).

Kitwood T. (1997). *Dementia Reconsidered: The Person Comes First*. Buckingham: Open University Press.

Kübler-Ross E. (1969). *On Death and Dying*. London: Routledge.

Leadership Alliance for the Care of Dying People. (2014). One chance to get it right. Available at: https://www.gov.uk/government/uploads/system/uploads/attachment_data/file/323188/One_chance_to_get_it_right.pdf (accessed on 28 October 2014).

McNamara N. (2014). Norms pages (Blog). Available at: http://tdaa.co.uk/norms-pages/ (accessed on 14 November 2014).

Mental Capacity Act. (2005). London: HMSO. Available at: http://www.legislation.gov.uk/ukpga/2005/9/contents (accessed on 14 November 2014).

Nasreddine ZS, Phillips NA, Bédirian V, Charbonneau S, Whitehead V, Collin I, Cummings JL, Chertkow H. (2005). The Montreal Cognitive Assessment, MoCA: a brief screening tool for mild cognitive impairment. *Journal of the American Geriatric Society*, 53(4), 695–699.

Nolan M. (2006). *The Senses Framework – Improving Care for Older People Through a Relationship-Centred Approach*. Sheffield: University of Sheffield.

Prasher V. (2005) *Alzheimer's Disease and Dementia in Down Syndrome and Intellectual Disabilities*. Oxford: Radcliffe.

Schweitzer P, Bruce E. (2008). *Remembering Yesterday, Caring Today: Reminiscence in Dementia Care*. London: Jessica Kingsley Publishers.

Scottish Executive. (2000). *Adults with Incapacity (Scotland) Act 2000*. Edinburgh: Stationery Office.

The Clear Communication People Ltd. (2013). The hospital communication booklet. Available at: www.communicationpeople.co.uk (accessed on 14 November 2014).

The Equality Act. (2010). London: HMSO. Available at: http://www.legislation.gov.uk/ukpga/2010/15/contents (accessed on 14 November 2014).

Tuppen J. (2012). The benefits of groups that provide cognitive stimulation for people with dementia. *Nursing Older People*, 24(10), 20–24.

Waterlow J. (2005). The waterlow score assessment tool. Available at: http://www.judy-waterlow.co.uk/waterlow_score.htm (accessed on 31 January 2014).

WHO. (n.d.). Pain relief ladder for cancer pain relief. Available at: www.who.int/cancer/palliative/painladder/en/ (accessed on 14 November 2014).

Woods B, Aguirre E, Spector AE, Orrell M. (2012). Cognitive stimulation to improve cognitive functioning in people with dementia. *Cochrane Database of Systematic Reviews*, (2), CD005562. DOI: 10.1002/14651858.CD005562.pub2.

Recommended Reading

Age UK. (2010). *Still Hungry to Be Heard: The Scandal of People in Later Life Becoming Malnourished in Hospital*. London: Age UK.

Alzheimer's Society. (2014). Dementia 2014 infographic. Available at: http://www.alzheimers.org.uk/infographic (accessed on 14 November 2014).

Anderson P. (2014). Getting the priorities right in end-of-life care. *Nursing Times*, 110(32–33), 19–20.

Banerjee S. (2010). *The Use of Antipsychotic Medication for People with Dementia: A Call for Action*. London: Department of Health.

Block S. (2009). *The Story of Forgetting*. London: Faber & Faber.

Brooker D. (2007). *Person Centred Dementia Care: Making Services Better*. London: Jessica Kingsley Publishers.

Bryden C. (2005). *Dancing with Dementia: My Story of Living Positively with Dementia*. London: Jessica Kingsley Publishers.

Dementia Services Development Centre. (2008). *Continence and People with Dementia*. Stirling: DSDC University of Stirling.

Dementia Services Development Centre. (2009). *Food and Nutrition for People with Dementia*. Stirling: DSDC University of Stirling.

Dementia Services Development Centre. (2012). *Design Features to Assist Patients with Dementia in General Hospitals and Emergency Departments*. Stirling: DSDC University of Stirling.

Downs M, Bowers B (eds.). (2014). *Excellence in Dementia Care: Research into Practice*, 2nd edition. Maidenhead: Open University Press.

Feil N. (2012). *The Validation Breakthrough: Simple Techniques for Communicating with People with Alzheimer's and Other Dementias*. Baltimore: Health Professions Press.

Genova L. (2012). *Still Alice*. London: Simon & Schuster.

Hindle A, Coates A (eds.). (2011). *Nursing Care of Older People: A Textbook for Students and Nurses*. Oxford: Oxford University Press.

Jenkins C, Smythe A. (2013). Reflections on a visit to a dementia care village. *Nursing Older People*, 25(6), 14–19.

Kelly F, Innes A. (2010). *End of Life Care for People with Dementia: A Best Practice Guide*. Stirling: DSDC University of Stirling.

Khan F, Curtice M. (2011). Non-pharmacological management of behavioural symptoms of dementia. *British Journal of Community Nursing*, 16(9), 441–449.

Killick J. (2008). *You Are Words: Dementia Poems*. London: Hawker Publications.

Kitwood T. (1997). *Dementia Reconsidered: The Person Comes First*. Buckingham: Open University Press.

Knocker S. (2013). Home from home. *Nursing Standard*, 27(22), 20–21.

Kyle G. (2012). Medication management in older people with dementia. *Journal of Community Nursing*, 26(1), 31–34.

Larson E, Wang L. (2006). Exercise is associated with reduced risk for incident dementia among persons 65 years of age and older. *Annals of Internal Medicine*, 144(2), 72–81.

Linden D. (2011). *The Biology of Psychological Disorders*. Basingstoke: Palgrave Macmillan.

MacLullich AMJ, Ferguson KJ, Miller T, de Rooijc SEJA, Cunningham C. (2008). Unravelling the pathophysiology of delirium: a focus on the role of aberrant stress responses. *Journal of Psychosomatic Research*, 65(3), 229–238.

Nash M. (2014). *Physical Health and Well-being in Mental Health Nursing: Clinical Skills for Practice*. Maidenhead: Open University Press.

Nolan M. (2006). *The Senses Framework – Improving Care for Older People Through a Relationship-Centred Approach*. Sheffield: University of Sheffield.

Prasher V. (2005). *Alzheimer's Disease and Dementia in Down Syndrome and Intellectual Disabilities*. Oxford: Radcliffe.

Royal College of Nursing. (2013). *Safeguarding Vulnerable Adults*. London: RCN Publishing.

Sheard D. (2009). *Nurturing Emotions at Work in Dementia Care*. London: Alzheimer's Society.

Websites

Action on Hearing Loss. (2010). Hearing matters. Available at: http://www.actiononhearingloss.org.uk/supporting-you/policy-research-and-influencing/research/hearing-matters.aspx (accessed on 14 November 2014).

Alzheimer's Society. Singing for the brain. Available at: http://www.alzheimers.org.uk/site/scripts/documents_info.php?documentID=760 (accessed on 14 November 2014).

Alzheimer's Society. (2013). Assistive technology – devices to help with everyday living. Factsheet 437LP. Available at: http://www.google.co.uk/url?sa=t&rct=j&q=&esrc=s&frm=1&source=web&cd=1&ved=0CDEQFjAA&url=http%3A%2F%2Fwww.alzheimers.org.uk%2Fsite%2Fscripts%2Fdownload.php%3FfileID%3D1779&ei=OLVkVI_6GILpaubMgfAO&usg=AFQjCNHkWzemsIxuDzYKRUfiyYKfbhWcsg (accessed on 14 November 2014).

British Geriatric Society guidelines for the prevention. (2006). Guidelines for the prevention, diagnosis and management of delirium in older people in hospital. Available at: http://www.bgs.org.uk/index.php/clinicalguides/170-clinguidedeliriumtreatment (accessed on 14 November 2014).

Dementia Services Development Centre. (2012). Virtual Care Home. Available at: www.dementia.stir.ac.uk/virtualhome (accessed on 14 November 2014).

Action on hearing lossNational Institute for Health and Care Excellence. (2006). Guideline CG32. Nutrition support in adults: Oral nutrition support, enteral tube feeding and parenteral nutrition. Available at: http://www.nice.org.uk/guidance/CG32 (accessed on 14 November 2014).

National Institute for Health and Care Excellence. (2006). Guideline CG42. Dementia: Supporting people with dementia and their carers in health and social care. Available at: http://www.nice.org.uk/guidance/CG42 (accessed on 14 November 2014).

National Institute for Health and Care Excellence. (2010). Guideline CG103. Delirium: Diagnosis, prevention and management. Available at: http://www.nice.org.uk/guidance/CG103 (accessed on 14 November 2014).

National Institute for Health and Care Excellence. (2011). Guideline QS13. Quality standard for end of life care for adults. Available at: https://www.nice.org.uk/guidance/QS13 (accessed on 13 November 2014).

National Institute for Health and Care Excellence. (2013). Guideline CG161. Falls: Assessment and prevention of falls in older people. Available at: https://www.nice.org.uk/guidance/cg161 (accessed on 14 November 2014).

National Institute for Health and Care Excellence. (2013). Guideline CG171. Urinary incontinence: The management of urinary incontinence in women. Available at: https://www.nice.org.uk/guidance/cg171 (accessed on 14 November 2014).

National Institute for Health and Care Excellence. (2013). Clinical knowledge summary. Available at: http://cks.nice.org.uk/constipation#!scenariorecommendation:5 (accessed on 14 November 2014).

National Institute for Health and Care Excellence. (2014). Guideline CG179. Pressure ulcers: Prevention and management of pressure ulcers. Available at: http://www.nice.org.uk/guidance/cg179 (accessed on 13 November 2014).

The Irish Hospice Foundation. (2013). Planning for the future project: Initiating 'End of Life' discussions for people with dementia. Available at: http://hospicefoundation.ie/wp-content/uploads/2014/03/Final-Report.pdf (accessed on 13 November 2014).

Index

Dementia Care at a Glance, First Edition. Catharine Jenkins, Laura Ginesi and Bernie Keenan. © 2016 by John Wiley & Sons, Ltd. Published 2016 by John Wiley & Sons, Ltd.
Companion website: www.ataglanceseries.com/nursing/dementiacare